LIFE ALCHEMY
1.0

THE DAILY WORKBOOK TO
IMPRESSIVELY TRANSFORM YOUR LIFE

Dr. Dale Ellwein

Life Alchemy 1.0: The Daily Workbook to Impressively Transform Your Life.

Copyright © 2014 by Dr. Dale Ellwein.

All rights reserved. Printed in the United States of America. No parts of this book may be used or reproduced in any manner whatsoever without written permission, except in the case of brief quotations embodied in critical articles and reviews. For information, address Dr. Dale Ellwein; 3436 N. Verdugo Rd., Suite 250, Glendale, CA 91208.

This book may be purchased for educational, business, or sales promotional use. For information please write: Dr. Dale Ellwein, 3436 N. Verdugo Rd., Suite 250, Glendale, CA 91208.

Life Alchemy 1.0 website: www.standingtallpublishing.com

Discounts for Bulk Sales are Available

Each of us has a sense of something possible beyond the ordinary. Each of us has moments when something about our lives, our family, our community, our world awakens in us a sense of possibility. Each of us has glimpses of that most fundamental of all possibilities - that life really could be extraordinary.

B.J. Palmer

NAME	_____
PHONE	_____
ADDRESS	_____
	_____
START DATE	_____
COMPLETION	_____

PREFACE

Ancient Alchemists were interested in transmutation, in other words, changing one thing into another. The most common thing people think of when they hear "alchemy" is the process of turning lead into gold. What *Life Alchemy 1.0* is about is turning your life into gold.

Using the language of the alchemists, there is a magical elixir that when administered, can truly, impressively transform your life. I have searched far and wide, sat at the feet of the masters, hunted through the ancient writings and manuscripts to uncover the keys to the Alchemy of Life for you. This is the key that will turn the ethers* that surround you into the solid life of your dreams.

As you step through this book, you will learn the art that is the Alchemy of Life. This dream that you envision can be, I dare say will be, yours as you learn to implement and synthesize these special formulas into your life. Out of the ethers, your life will be made clear in vision and then in form as you proceed and make a habit of these sacred steps.

Awaken to your inner power! Take action and transform your life now.

*Ether: There are four physical elements that describe the material Universe. But ether, the fifth element, describes the Spirit that exists beyond matter. – *Akash and the Book of Life* by Ervin Laszlo, Ph.D.

INTRODUCTION

Here's How It Works...

Each day you will start with your Daily Preview, and at the end of the day, your Daily Review. Your Daily Preview is all about setting up your day. It is for focusing, building energy, and creating your day as it begins. Ideally, this part should be done within the first few minutes after arising. It should go something like this...

The alarm goes off, you shut it off, you get up (no more snooze button!), you go to the bathroom, you start your coffee or tea, sit, take a breath, grab your workbook and get to it.

It should only take about 5 - 10 minutes, but if you feel like adding affirmations, meditation, prayer, exercise, or reading something inspirational to your morning routine, go for it. I highly recommend this, but if you only have a few minutes, just grab the workbook.

Your Daily Review should be done at the end of the day—either right after your workday or right before you go to bed—whichever works best for you.

The purpose of your Daily Review is to check in with yourself. See how your day was. See if there were any wins or things you need to improve that came up for you. It is mostly an opportunity for you to hold yourself accountable and learn some things about yourself.

For added accountability, enlist the help of a friend, your spouse, or your health partner. They may wish to participate with you or maybe you can just ask them to ask you, "How's your life alchemy going?"

The First 6 Days

During the first 6 days of this 91 day program, you will be doing some exercises to help you establish a focus, as well as help you develop habits that will transform your life. As you go through this process, you will set goals, establish a vision of your ideal life, nail down some habits that must be implemented and/or eliminated, and learn how to use this workbook to really create the positive changes necessary to set yourself up to win in life.

In order to separate the core of the workbook from the direction over the first 6 days, my guidance will all be italicized.

Hang in there. We will take this one step at a time and after 91 days, I predict you will be so thrilled that you will want to continue doing this process for the rest of your life.

> *"When eating an elephant take one bite at a time."*
>
> *Creighton Abrams*

LET'S TAKE THAT FIRST BITE. TURN THE PAGE TO DAY 1.

DAILY PREVIEW
DAY 1

M T W T F S S

Date: _____

In the workbook, you will notice Day 1, Day 2, etc. This goes up to Day 91 and marks off your 91 day program.

Your first assignment is easy. Circle the letter that represents the day of the week and fill in the dates for the first seven days. For the highly committed, write it in pen. For those who may not be able to be fully committed, write in pencil. Filling in each box reinforces your intention to commit to this program.

Done the assignment? Awesome! You are on your way!

As you went through your workbook numbering the dates, you may have noticed that on every day, there is a list of Action Steps for that day. As we go through these first 6 days, you will develop your vision of an ideal situation for your life and you will set some goals. With those in mind, you can choose actions to achieve them and put them into your daily Action Steps for Today. By defining your goals and regularly taking steps towards them, you will eventually get the life of your dreams.

"A journey of a thousand miles begins with a single step."

Lao-Tzu

Take a moment and write some of the Actions Steps for Today. The High Priority steps should be reserved for the things that are most important in your life. Medium Priority describes the things that are slightly less important. Low Priority describes the least vital actions needed that day.

As you complete the Action Steps, check them off. Remember to glance at this list as you go through your day. This way you won't miss the important actions that are getting you where you ultimately want to go. If you do not wish to carry around your workbook, you can take a picture of your Daily Preview with your smart phone and look at it throughout the day.

If, in the morning you have a thought or a flash of genius, capture it in your Morning Thoughts and Inspirations box.

→

Each day there will be a box offered to you to do just that.

Remember, tonight you will be reviewing how you did with your action steps. This will help with your personal accountability and allow you to create the life of your dreams. Go make your day amazing!

ACTION STEPS FOR TODAY

High Priority
1. _____
2. _____
3. _____

Medium Priority
1. _____
2. _____
3. _____

Low Priority
_____
_____
_____
_____
_____
_____
_____

MORNING THOUGHTS AND INSPIRATIONS

DAILY REVIEW DAY 1

Every day, you will notice as part of your Daily Review this section "Today I am Grateful for..."

Today I am grateful for...

_____
_____
_____
_____
_____
_____
_____
_____

A Quick Word on Gratitude

Along with love, gratitude is one of the most powerful feelings that you can have on a regular basis. Think about it. If someone is truly grateful for what you have given them, will you be more likely to give them more? Is a person in a state of gratitude more satisfied and happy in life? Of course! Therefore it is imperative for you to develop a genuine attitude of gratitude so you can really live in the joy of life.

Throughout your day, notice some things that you are grateful for and either write them down right away, or write them during your Daily Review. By doing this every day, you will develop the habit of looking for things to be grateful for.

Self-Accountability

Ultimately, in life, you are the most important person to be accountable to. Sure, you can hire a coach, or enlist a friend or your spouse to help you stay accountable, but really, it's up to you whether you will follow through on something or not. This is what this section is about. It's a self-check. It can be an "attaboy" or "attagirl", or it can be a course correction.

How was my day? Did I feel good about my performance? What did I learn? Did I have a new insight? What would I do differently?

_____
_____
_____
_____
_____

You get to decide how to best use this section, but make sure you take advantage of it. At the end of the week, you can review this area and get an overview of how everything is going for you.

Congratulations! You have made it through Day 1. Be proud of yourself and celebrate! See you tomorrow.

Life Alchemy 1.0

DAILY PREVIEW
DAY 2

M T W T F S S

Date: _____

My Primary Objective
_____
_____

Between where you are and where you would like to be, there is a gap. There is a technology to bridging that gap so you can have the life you want. This is the alchemy that this workbook is all about: helping you to become the person that can easily have all that you want in life. The first step is to know what you want. If you can really define your target, you can more easily hit it. Let's have some fun! Answer this question, and let your mind go wild.

If there were no rules, and I could not fail, what would my life be like? Describe this future life in detail and in writing.

ACTION STEPS FOR TODAY

High Priority
1. _____
2. _____
3. _____

Medium Priority
1. _____
2. _____
3. _____

Low Priority
_____
_____
_____
_____
_____
_____

Look through your future life. Feels pretty good, doesn't it? Now, fill in the blank...

If I only accomplish _____, my future life would surely come to be.

Whatever single thing you write in the above box you can use as your Primary Objective throughout this book. My intention for you is that you either move closer to achieving your Primary Objective, or you get it, in the next 3 months. The next question to answer is: What do you suppose it would feel like if you achieved your Primary Objective? Describe how it would feel as if you have accomplished it now.

This is the big formula in the alchemy of life: know what you want, visualize it as if it has come to be, and feel it as if it has been accomplished. Of course, now you must take action towards its completion. Write your Primary Objective in the box above and set your Action Steps for Today. Be sure to include at least one thing in your High Priority list that you can do today that will get you a step closer to your future ideal life.

DAILY REVIEW DAY 2

How was your day? Did you accomplish your highest priority action steps? Are you feeling more energy throughout your day? Are you excited about what tomorrow will bring? These are some of the things to write in your "notes and reflections from today box."

Take some time to review and reflect on your day.

Today I am grateful for...

_____
_____
_____
_____
_____
_____
_____
_____

How was my day? Did I feel good about my performance? What did I learn? Did I have a new insight? What would I do differently?

_____
_____
_____
_____
_____
_____
_____
_____

NOTES AND REFLECTIONS FROM TODAY

If you have filled in the above boxes, you're doing great! Now take a look below. Is there anything you can think of for tomorrow? Did you miss an action step? Is there an action step that you want to put down and get out of your mind?

If there is anything on your mind about tomorrow, put it in there. Also, take a moment and read a daily quote, too. Sleep well. See you tomorrow.

FOR TOMORROW

_____
_____
_____
_____

"All you need is the plan, the road map, and the courage to press on to your destination."

— Earl Nightingale

DAILY PREVIEW
DAY 3

M T W T F S S

Date: _____

Welcome to Day 3! Do you remember your Primary Objective that you put together yesterday? Every day, you will be taking a moment to write it down. There is something magical that happens when you write down something that you want in life. It is like the Universe takes you more seriously and delivers it to you faster. So, write down your Primary Objective daily, and watch what happens!

MY PRIMARY OBJECTIVE

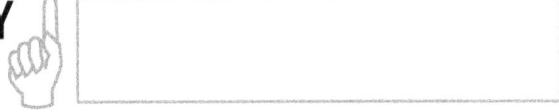

One way to help you open up to possibilities is a technique called sentence completion. Every day, you will be completing sentences to help you determine your best course of action for getting closer to your Primary Objective.

Complete these sentences. The only rule is to not repeat your answer.

The most important thing I can do today to take me a step closer to my Primary Objective is _____.

The most important thing I can do today to take me a step closer to my Primary Objective is _____.

The most important thing I can do today to take me a step closer to my Primary Objective is _____.

The most important thing I can do today to take me a step closer to my Primary Objective is _____.

Now, take one or more of those answers and place it (them) in the High Priority Action Steps for Today list.

Can you see how if you take at least one step a day towards your future life you will eventually arrive there?

Now, some of these Actions Steps may be easy, and some may be more challenging. Tomorrow we will give you a strategy to help you with the more challenging ones.

ACTION STEPS FOR TODAY

High Priority
1. _____
2. _____
3. _____

Medium Priority
1. _____
2. _____
3. _____

Low Priority
_____
_____
_____
_____
_____
_____

MORNING THOUGHTS AND INSPIRATIONS

DAILY REVIEW
DAY 3

Do you see how each day is building on the last? Do you notice how you are actually moving in the direction of your future? Are you noticing any internal resistance?

Fill in your Daily Review.

Today I am grateful for...

_____
_____
_____
_____
_____
_____
_____
_____

How was my day? Did I feel good about my performance? What did I learn? Did I have a new insight? What would I do differently?

_____
_____
_____
_____
_____
_____
_____
_____

NOTES AND REFLECTIONS FROM TODAY

Let's check in on your energy for the day. Energy is what allows you to charge ahead and get things done. It is the spark of life. Every day you will gauge your energy because you can only change things when you become aware of them.

What was my energy level today? (lowest to highest) 1 2 3 4 5 6 7 8 9 10

If not a "10", what will I do tomorrow to make it closer to a "10"? _____

FOR TOMORROW

_____
_____
_____
_____

"The key to success is to focus our conscious mind on things we desire, not things we fear."

Brian Tracy

DAILY PREVIEW
DAY 4

M T W T F S S

Date: _____

MY PRIMARY OBJECTIVE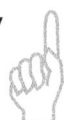

[_____]

The most important thing I can do today to take me a step closer to my Primary Objective is _____.

The most important thing I can do today to take me a step closer to my Primary Objective is _____.

The most important thing I can do today to take me a step closer to my Primary Objective is _____.

The most important thing I can do today to take me a step closer to my Primary Objective is _____.

Eat that Frog

"Eat a live frog first thing in the morning and nothing worse will happen to you the rest of the day."

— Mark Twain

A live frog is the thing that you know you should do and maybe need to do, but you are just not doing it. Maybe it's a phone call. Maybe it is approaching someone or confronting an issue that needs to be handled. It could be something you feel afraid of, but once you do it, you feel energized and super!

So, if you can eat the biggest, ugliest frog first thing in the day, the rest of the day will be much easier. This is an amazing habit to create. It will stretch you and help you grow into the future you desire. Have you noticed yet that sometimes your greatest successes lay right on the other side of your fears?

Complete this statement... and eat that frog!

Something I have been putting off that I know would be great if I did it is...

_____

ACTION STEPS FOR TODAY

High Priority

1. _____
2. _____
3. _____

Medium Priority

1. _____
2. _____
3. _____

Low Priority

_____
_____
_____
_____
_____
_____

MORNING THOUGHTS AND INSPIRATIONS

How did you do with that frog? If you would define a frog to eat every day and eat it, can you see how empowering that will be for you? You are building your fear-busting muscle; you're becoming unstoppable!

DAILY REVIEW
DAY 4

Today I am grateful for...

_____
_____
_____
_____
_____
_____
_____
_____

How was my day? Did I feel good about my performance? What did I learn? Did I have a new insight? What would I do differently?

_____
_____
_____
_____
_____
_____
_____
_____

NOTES AND REFLECTIONS FROM TODAY

What was my energy level today? (lowest to highest)   1 2 3 4 5 6 7 8 9 10

If not a "10", what will I do tomorrow to make it closer to a "10"? _____

Here is your Frog Eating accountability space. Every day note whether or not you ate your frog and what time. We'll take a look at this in the weekly review.

I ate my frog today: Yes   No

What Time? _____

FOR TOMORROW

_____
_____
_____
_____
_____

"Courage is the commitment to begin without any guarantee of success."
Johann Wolfgang von Goethe

Life Alchemy 1.0

DAILY PREVIEW
DAY 5

M T W T F S S

Date: _____

MY PRIMARY OBJECTIVE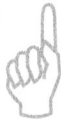

[_____]

The most important thing I can do today to take me a step closer to my Primary Objective is _____.

The most important thing I can do today to take me a step closer to my Primary Objective is _____.

The most important thing I can do today to take me a step closer to my Primary Objective is _____.

The most important thing I can do today to take me a step closer to my Primary Objective is _____.

What you habitually think about and act upon determines your destiny. In other words, if you change your habits, you change your life.

"Insanity: doing the same thing over and over again and expecting different results."
— Albert Einstein

It takes about 28 days to establish a new habit. Since this book is split into three 28-day sections, by the end, you will have established 3 new, life-changing habits!

You get a choice here. You can either add a new good habit (like doing your workbook everyday), or you can eliminate a bad habit. So fill in the blank...

If I consistently did _____,
I know that I would get my Primary Objective.

Or if I quit doing _____,
I know that I would get my Primary Objective.

My new habit I'm developing (or eliminating) is...
_____
_____

My biggest frog to eat today...
_____

ACTION STEPS FOR TODAY

High Priority
1. _____
2. _____
3. _____

Medium Priority
1. _____
2. _____
3. _____

Low Priority
_____
_____
_____
_____
_____
_____

MORNING THOUGHTS AND INSPIRATIONS

DAILY REVIEW
DAY 5

You may notice a new piece of the puzzle at the bottom of this page. It is a check-in about your new habit.

I am really proud of you. As you continue this process, take the time to notice how your life is transforming.

Today I am grateful for...

_____
_____
_____
_____
_____
_____
_____
_____

How was my day? Did I feel good about my performance? What did I learn? Did I have a new insight? What would I do differently?

_____
_____
_____
_____
_____
_____
_____
_____

NOTES AND REFLECTIONS FROM TODAY

What was my energy level today? (lowest to highest) 1 2 3 4 5 6 7 8 9 10

If not a "10", what will I do tomorrow to make it closer to a "10"? _____

I ate my frog today: Yes   No   I did my new habit: Yes   No

What Time? _____   What Time? _____

FOR TOMORROW

_____
_____
_____
_____

"Success seems to be largely a matter of hanging on after others have let go."
William Feather

Life Alchemy 1.0

DAILY PREVIEW
DAY 6

M T W T F S S

Date: _____

My biggest frog to eat today...
_____

ACTION STEPS FOR TODAY

MY PRIMARY OBJECTIVE

The most important thing I can do today to take me a step closer to my Primary Objective is _____.

The most important thing I can do today to take me a step closer to my Primary Objective is _____.

The most important thing I can do today to take me a step closer to my Primary Objective is _____.

The most important thing I can do today to take me a step closer to my Primary Objective is _____.

My new habit I'm developing (eliminating) is... _____

Balance in life creates a fuller, more whole life experience. Below are 7 key areas of life. Rank yourself on a 1 (poor) to 10 (optimum) scale to get an idea of how balanced (or out of balance) your life is.

Every day, you will get a chance to focus on one or more of these areas.

Physical Health	1	2	3	4	5	6	7	8	9	10
Financial Health	1	2	3	4	5	6	7	8	9	10
Family Health	1	2	3	4	5	6	7	8	9	10
Social Health	1	2	3	4	5	6	7	8	9	10
Career Health	1	2	3	4	5	6	7	8	9	10
Spiritual Health	1	2	3	4	5	6	7	8	9	10
Mental Health	1	2	3	4	5	6	7	8	9	10

High Priority
1. _____
2. _____
3. _____

Medium Priority
1. _____
2. _____
3. _____

Low Priority
_____
_____
_____
_____
_____
_____

MORNING THOUGHTS AND INSPIRATIONS

DAILY REVIEW
DAY 6

Weekly Goal Focus:

Every week, pick a goal that inspires you and takes you closer to your ideal life. When you regularly focus on a goal, it makes it easier for you to recognize when the opportunities appear for you to take action towards that goal. This Weekly Goal can be your Primary Objective, or something even bigger.

Today I am grateful for...

___

How was my day? Did I feel good about my performance? What did I learn? Did I have a new insight? What would I do differently?

___

NOTES AND REFLECTIONS FROM TODAY

What was my energy level today? (lowest to highest) 1 2 3 4 5 6 7 8 9 10

If not a "10", what will I do tomorrow to make it closer to a "10"? _____

I ate my frog today: Yes No

What Time? _____

I did my new habit: Yes No

What Time? _____

FOR TOMORROW

___

"You never know how far reaching something you think, say, or do today, will affect the lives of millions tomorrow."

B.J Palmer

Life Alchemy 1.0

DAILY PREVIEW
DAY 7

M T W T F S S

Date: _____

MY PRIMARY OBJECTIVE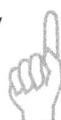

[_____]

The most important thing I can do today to take me a step closer to my Primary Objective is _____.

The most important thing I can do today to take me a step closer to my Primary Objective is _____.

The most important thing I can do today to take me a step closer to my Primary Objective is _____.

The most important thing I can do today to take me a step closer to my Primary Objective is _____.

My new habit I'm developing (eliminating) is... _____

MORNING THOUGHTS AND INSPIRATIONS

My biggest frog to eat today...
_____

ACTION STEPS FOR TODAY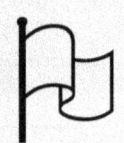

High Priority
1. _____
2. _____
3. _____

Medium Priority
1. _____
2. _____
3. _____

Low Priority
_____
_____
_____
_____
_____
_____

In which area(s) do I want to improve the most today?

Mental Health

Spiritual Health

Career Health

Physical Health

Social Health

Family Health

Financial Health

Weekly Goal Focus:

DAILY REVIEW
DAY 7

Today I am grateful for...

_____
_____
_____
_____
_____
_____
_____

How was my day? Did I feel good about my performance? What did I learn? Did I have a new insight? What would I do differently?

_____
_____
_____
_____
_____
_____
_____

NOTES AND REFLECTIONS FROM TODAY

What was my energy level today? (lowest to highest) 1 2 3 4 5 6 7 8 9 10

If not a "10", what will I do tomorrow to make it closer to a "10"? _____

I ate my frog today: Yes   No

What Time? _____

I did my new habit: Yes   No

What Time? _____

FOR TOMORROW

_____
_____
_____
_____

"Action is the foundational key to all success."

Pablo Picasso

Life Alchemy 1.0

WEEKLY CHECK-IN
WEEK 1

The Purpose of the Weekly Check-In is to...

1) Check-in with your progress throughout the week.

2) Re-focus for the upcoming week.

3) Get inspired for the future.

THE CHECK-IN

What have I accomplished since last week? What were the two most important things that I learned this week? Is there anything that I would have done differently? If so, what?

_____
_____
_____
_____

What are my wins or victories since last week?

_____
_____
_____

What's the highlight (or low-light) of my week?

_____
_____
_____

What am I thankful for this week?

_____
_____
_____

The place I feel stuck is

_____
_____
_____

In which area(s) did I grow the most last week?

Mental Health

Spiritual Health

Career Health

Physical Health

Social Health

Family Health

Financial Health

What was my average energy level for the week?

1 2 3 4 5 6 7 8 9 10

What number do I want it to be next week?

1 2 3 4 5 6 7 8 9 10

How often did you eat your frog?

1 2 3 4 (Next week you'll have 7 opportunities)

On a 1 - 10 scale, 1 being low and 10 being high, how grateful have I been feeling this last week?

1 2 3 4 5 6 7 8 9 10

How did I do with my new habit building/eliminating?

_____
_____
_____

Every week, we will be re-focusing on our future life. So, take a moment and fill this in again. There will be a few questions after you finish.

RE-FOCUS
WEEK 1

If there were no rules, and I could not fail, what would my life be like?

Describe your future life in detail and in writing...

_____
_____
_____
_____
_____
_____
_____

When you wrote this out again, how did you feel? Were you excited? Were you bored? Did your vision evolve? Was it different than before? Was there more detail or less? Did you even do this exercise? If not, how come?

_____
_____
_____

Set Your Primary Objective for next week.

Look through your future life. Now, fill in the blank...

If I only accomplish _____ next week, my future life would surely come to be.

This is your Primary Objective for the next week.

(As a special note, if by chance you miss a few days or stray from the process of working in this book on a daily basis, when you are ready to get started again, go to the next Weekly Check-In section and start there. This is an excellent place to jump back in and get going again.)

Take a moment and fill in the days of the week for the next week.

Go on to Day 8 and be amazing!

Life Alchemy 1.0

DAILY PREVIEW
DAY 8

M T W T F S S

Date: _____

MY PRIMARY OBJECTIVE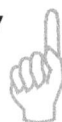

[   ]

The most important thing I can do today to take me a step closer to my Primary Objective is _____ .

The most important thing I can do today to take me a step closer to my Primary Objective is _____ .

The most important thing I can do today to take me a step closer to my Primary Objective is _____ .

The most important thing I can do today to take me a step closer to my Primary Objective is _____ .

My new habit I'm developing (eliminating) is... _____

MORNING THOUGHTS AND INSPIRATIONS

My biggest frog to eat today...
_____

ACTION STEPS FOR TODAY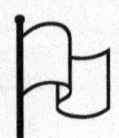

High Priority
1. _____
2. _____
3. _____

Medium Priority
1. _____
2. _____
3. _____

Low Priority
_____
_____
_____
_____
_____
_____

In which area(s) do I want to improve the most today?

Mental Health

Spiritual Health

Career Health

Physical Health

Social Health

Family Health

Financial Health

Weekly Goal Focus:

DAILY REVIEW
DAY 8

Today I am grateful for...

_____
_____
_____
_____
_____
_____
_____

How was my day? Did I feel good about my performance? What did I learn? Did I have a new insight? What would I do differently?

_____
_____
_____
_____
_____
_____
_____

NOTES AND REFLECTIONS FROM TODAY

What was my energy level today? (lowest to highest)   1 2 3 4 5 6 7 8 9 10

If not a "10", what will I do tomorrow to make it closer to a "10"? _____

I ate my frog today: Yes   No   I did my new habit: Yes   No

What Time? _____   What Time? _____

FOR TOMORROW

_____
_____
_____
_____

"I honestly think it is better to be a failure at something you love than to be a success at something you hate."
— George Burns

Life Alchemy 1.0

DAILY PREVIEW
DAY 9

M T W T F S S

Date: _____

MY PRIMARY OBJECTIVE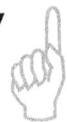

[_____]

The most important thing I can do today to take me a step closer to my Primary Objective is _____.

The most important thing I can do today to take me a step closer to my Primary Objective is _____.

The most important thing I can do today to take me a step closer to my Primary Objective is _____.

The most important thing I can do today to take me a step closer to my Primary Objective is _____.

My new habit I'm developing (eliminating) is... _____

MORNING THOUGHTS AND INSPIRATIONS

My biggest frog to eat today...
_____

ACTION STEPS FOR TODAY

High Priority
1. _____
2. _____
3. _____

Medium Priority
1. _____
2. _____
3. _____

Low Priority
_____
_____
_____
_____
_____
_____

In which area(s) do I want to improve the most today?

Mental Health

Spiritual Health

Career Health

Physical Health

Social Health

Family Health

Financial Health

Weekly Goal Focus:

DAILY REVIEW
DAY 9

Today I am grateful for...

_____
_____
_____
_____
_____
_____
_____
_____

How was my day? Did I feel good about my performance? What did I learn? Did I have a new insight? What would I do differently?

_____
_____
_____
_____
_____
_____
_____
_____

NOTES AND REFLECTIONS FROM TODAY

What was my energy level today? (lowest to highest) 1 2 3 4 5 6 7 8 9 10

If not a "10", what will I do tomorrow to make it closer to a "10"? _____

I ate my frog today: Yes   No

What Time? _____

I did my new habit: Yes   No

What Time? _____

FOR TOMORROW

_____
_____
_____
_____

"Success is getting what you want. Happiness is wanting what you get."
  — *Dale Carnegie*

Life Alchemy 1.0

DAILY PREVIEW
DAY 10

M T W T F S S

Date: _____

MY PRIMARY OBJECTIVE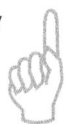

The most important thing I can do today to take me a step closer to my Primary Objective is _____.

The most important thing I can do today to take me a step closer to my Primary Objective is _____.

The most important thing I can do today to take me a step closer to my Primary Objective is _____.

The most important thing I can do today to take me a step closer to my Primary Objective is _____.

My new habit I'm developing (eliminating) is… _____

MORNING THOUGHTS AND INSPIRATIONS

My biggest frog to eat today…
_____

ACTION STEPS FOR TODAY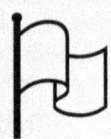

High Priority
1. _____
2. _____
3. _____

Medium Priority
1. _____
2. _____
3. _____

Low Priority
_____
_____
_____
_____
_____
_____

In which area(s) do I want to improve the most today?

Mental Health

Spiritual Health

Career Health

Physical Health

Social Health

Family Health

Financial Health

Weekly Goal Focus:

DAILY REVIEW
DAY 10

Today I am grateful for...

_____
_____
_____
_____
_____
_____
_____

How was my day? Did I feel good about my performance? What did I learn? Did I have a new insight? What would I do differently?

_____
_____
_____
_____
_____
_____
_____

NOTES AND REFLECTIONS FROM TODAY

What was my energy level today? (lowest to highest)   1 2 3 4 5 6 7 8 9 10

If not a "10", what will I do tomorrow to make it closer to a "10"? _____

I ate my frog today: Yes   No

What Time? _____

I did my new habit: Yes   No

What Time? _____

"The starting point of all achievement is desire."

Napoleon Hill

FOR TOMORROW

_____
_____
_____
_____

DAILY PREVIEW
DAY 11

M T W T F S S

Date: _____

MY PRIMARY OBJECTIVE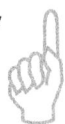

_____

The most important thing I can do today to take me a step closer to my Primary Objective is _____.

The most important thing I can do today to take me a step closer to my Primary Objective is _____.

The most important thing I can do today to take me a step closer to my Primary Objective is _____.

The most important thing I can do today to take me a step closer to my Primary Objective is _____.

My new habit I'm developing (eliminating) is… _____

MORNING THOUGHTS AND INSPIRATIONS

My biggest frog to eat today...
_____

ACTION STEPS FOR TODAY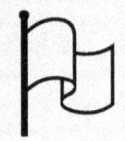

High Priority
1. _____
2. _____
3. _____

Medium Priority
1. _____
2. _____
3. _____

Low Priority
_____
_____
_____
_____
_____
_____

In which area(s) do I want to improve the most today?

- Mental Health
- Spiritual Health
- Career Health
- Physical Health
- Social Health
- Family Health
- Financial Health

Weekly Goal Focus:

DAILY REVIEW
DAY 11

Today I am grateful for...

_____
_____
_____
_____
_____
_____
_____
_____

How was my day? Did I feel good about my performance? What did I learn? Did I have a new insight? What would I do differently?

_____
_____
_____
_____
_____
_____
_____
_____

NOTES AND REFLECTIONS FROM TODAY

What was my energy level today? (lowest to highest) 1 2 3 4 5 6 7 8 9 10

If not a "10", what will I do tomorrow to make it closer to a "10"? _____

I ate my frog today: Yes   No   I did my new habit: Yes   No

What Time? _____   What Time? _____

FOR TOMORROW

_____
_____
_____
_____

"There is little success where there is little laughter."

Andrew Carnegie

Life Alchemy 1.0

DAILY PREVIEW
DAY 12

M T W T F S S

Date: _____

MY PRIMARY OBJECTIVE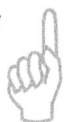

[_____]

The most important thing I can do today to take me a step closer to my Primary Objective is _____ .

The most important thing I can do today to take me a step closer to my Primary Objective is _____ .

The most important thing I can do today to take me a step closer to my Primary Objective is _____ .

The most important thing I can do today to take me a step closer to my Primary Objective is _____ .

My new habit I'm developing (eliminating) is... _____

MORNING THOUGHTS AND INSPIRATIONS

My biggest frog to eat today...
_____

ACTION STEPS FOR TODAY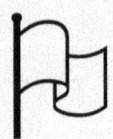

High Priority
1. _____
2. _____
3. _____

Medium Priority
1. _____
2. _____
3. _____

Low Priority
_____
_____
_____
_____
_____
_____

In which area(s) do I want to improve the most today?

Mental Health

Spiritual Health

Career Health

Physical Health

Social Health

Family Health

Financial Health

Weekly Goal Focus:

DAILY REVIEW
DAY 12

Today I am grateful for...

_____
_____
_____
_____
_____
_____
_____

How was my day? Did I feel good about my performance? What did I learn? Did I have a new insight? What would I do differently?

_____
_____
_____
_____
_____
_____
_____

NOTES AND REFLECTIONS FROM TODAY

What was my energy level today? (lowest to highest) 1 2 3 4 5 6 7 8 9 10

If not a "10", what will I do tomorrow to make it closer to a "10"? _____

I ate my frog today: Yes   No

What Time? _____

I did my new habit: Yes   No

What Time? _____

FOR TOMORROW

_____
_____
_____
_____

"Energy and persistence conquer all things."

Benjamin Franklin

Life Alchemy 1.0

DAILY PREVIEW
DAY 13

M T W T F S S

Date: _____

MY PRIMARY OBJECTIVE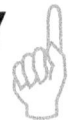

_____

The most important thing I can do today to take me a step closer to my Primary Objective is _____ .

The most important thing I can do today to take me a step closer to my Primary Objective is _____ .

The most important thing I can do today to take me a step closer to my Primary Objective is _____ .

The most important thing I can do today to take me a step closer to my Primary Objective is _____ .

My new habit I'm developing (eliminating) is... _____

MORNING THOUGHTS AND INSPIRATIONS

My biggest frog to eat today...
_____

ACTION STEPS FOR TODAY

High Priority
1. _____
2. _____
3. _____

Medium Priority
1. _____
2. _____
3. _____

Low Priority
_____
_____
_____
_____
_____
_____

In which area(s) do I want to improve the most today?

Mental Health

Spiritual Health

Career Health

Physical Health

Social Health

Family Health

Financial Health

Weekly Goal Focus:

DAILY REVIEW
DAY 13

Today I am grateful for...

_____
_____
_____
_____
_____
_____
_____

How was my day? Did I feel good about my performance? What did I learn? Did I have a new insight? What would I do differently?

_____
_____
_____
_____
_____
_____
_____

NOTES AND REFLECTIONS FROM TODAY

What was my energy level today? (lowest to highest) 1 2 3 4 5 6 7 8 9 10

If not a "10", what will I do tomorrow to make it closer to a "10"? _____

I ate my frog today: Yes   No

What Time? _____

I did my new habit: Yes   No

What Time? _____

FOR TOMORROW

_____
_____
_____
_____

"Today I will do what others won't, so tomorrow I can do what others can't."

Jerry Rice

Life Alchemy 1.0

DAILY PREVIEW
DAY 14

M T W T F S S

Date: _____

MY PRIMARY OBJECTIVE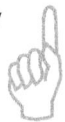

The most important thing I can do today to take me a step closer to my Primary Objective is _____.

The most important thing I can do today to take me a step closer to my Primary Objective is _____.

The most important thing I can do today to take me a step closer to my Primary Objective is _____.

The most important thing I can do today to take me a step closer to my Primary Objective is _____.

My new habit I'm developing (eliminating) is... _____

MORNING THOUGHTS AND INSPIRATIONS

My biggest frog to eat today...
_____

ACTION STEPS FOR TODAY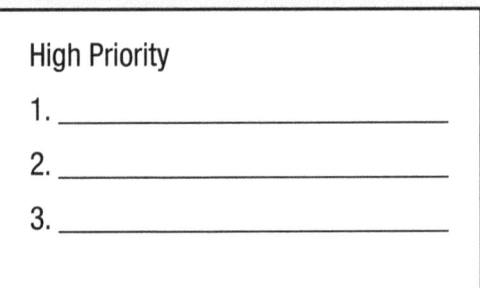

High Priority
1. _____
2. _____
3. _____

Medium Priority
1. _____
2. _____
3. _____

Low Priority
_____
_____
_____
_____
_____
_____

In which area(s) do I want to improve the most today?

Mental Health

Spiritual Health

Career Health

Physical Health

Social Health

Family Health

Financial Health

Weekly Goal Focus:

DAILY REVIEW
DAY 14

Today I am grateful for...

_____
_____
_____
_____
_____
_____
_____

How was my day? Did I feel good about my performance? What did I learn? Did I have a new insight? What would I do differently?

_____
_____
_____
_____
_____
_____
_____

NOTES AND REFLECTIONS FROM TODAY

What was my energy level today? (lowest to highest)   1 2 3 4 5 6 7 8 9 10

If not a "10", what will I do tomorrow to make it closer to a "10"? _____

I ate my frog today: Yes   No

What Time? _____

I did my new habit: Yes   No

What Time? _____

FOR TOMORROW

_____
_____
_____
_____

"Don't let the noise of other's opinions drown out your own inner voice."
                                            Steve Jobs

Life Alchemy 1.0

WEEKLY CHECK-INS
WEEK 2

The Purpose of the Weekly Check-In is to...

1) Check-in with your progress throughout the week.

2) Re-focus for the upcoming week.

3) Get inspired for the future.

THE CHECK-IN

What have I accomplished since last week? What were the two most important things that I learned this week? Is there anything that I would have done differently? If so, what?

___
___
___
___
___

What are my wins or victories since last week?

___
___
___

What's the highlight (or low-light) of my week?

___
___
___

What am I thankful for this week?

___
___
___

The place I feel stuck is

___
___
___

In which area(s) did I grow the most last week?

Mental Health

Spiritual Health

Career Health

Physical Health

Social Health

Family Health

Financial Health

What was my average energy level for the week?

1 2 3 4 5 6 7 8 9 10

What number do I want it to be next week?

1 2 3 4 5 6 7 8 9 10

How often did you eat your frog?

1 2 3 4 5 6 7

On a 1 - 10 scale, 1 being low and 10 being high, how grateful have I been feeling this last week?

1 2 3 4 5 6 7 8 9 10

How did I do with my new habit building/eliminating?

___
___
___

Every week, we will be re-focusing on our future life. So, take a moment and fill this in again. There will be a few questions after you finish.

RE-FOCUS
WEEK 2

If there were no rules, and I could not fail, what would my life be like?

Describe your future life in detail and in writing...

_____
_____
_____
_____
_____
_____
_____

When you wrote this out again, how did you feel? Were you excited? Were you bored? Did your vision evolve? Was it different than before? Was there more detail or less? Did you even do this exercise? If not, how come?

_____
_____
_____

Look through your future life. Now, fill in the blank...

If I only accomplish _____ next week, my future life would surely come to be.

This is your Primary Objective for the next week.

Take a moment and fill in the days of the week for the next week.

Go on to Day 15 and be amazing!

Life Alchemy 1.0

DAILY PREVIEW
DAY 15

M T W T F S S

Date: _____

MY PRIMARY OBJECTIVE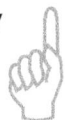

[_____]

The most important thing I can do today to take me a step closer to my Primary Objective is _____.

The most important thing I can do today to take me a step closer to my Primary Objective is _____.

The most important thing I can do today to take me a step closer to my Primary Objective is _____.

The most important thing I can do today to take me a step closer to my Primary Objective is _____.

My new habit I'm developing (eliminating) is... _____

MORNING THOUGHTS AND INSPIRATIONS

My biggest frog to eat today...
_____

ACTION STEPS FOR TODAY 🚩

High Priority
1. _____
2. _____
3. _____

Medium Priority
1. _____
2. _____
3. _____

Low Priority
_____
_____
_____
_____
_____
_____

In which area(s) do I want to improve the most today?

Mental Health

Spiritual Health

Career Health

Physical Health

Social Health

Family Health

Financial Health

Weekly Goal Focus:

DAILY REVIEW
DAY 15

Today I am grateful for...

How was my day? Did I feel good about my performance? What did I learn? Did I have a new insight? What would I do differently?

NOTES AND REFLECTIONS FROM TODAY

What was my energy level today? (lowest to highest)   1 2 3 4 5 6 7 8 9 10

If not a "10", what will I do tomorrow to make it closer to a "10"? _____

I ate my frog today: Yes   No   I did my new habit: Yes   No

What Time? _____   What Time? _____

FOR TOMORROW

"Anytime you stop striving to get better, you're bound to get worse."

Pat Riley

DAILY PREVIEW
DAY 16

M T W T F S S

Date: _____

MY PRIMARY OBJECTIVE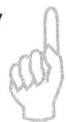

[_____]

The most important thing I can do today to take me a step closer to my Primary Objective is _____ .

The most important thing I can do today to take me a step closer to my Primary Objective is _____ .

The most important thing I can do today to take me a step closer to my Primary Objective is _____ .

The most important thing I can do today to take me a step closer to my Primary Objective is _____ .

My new habit I'm developing (eliminating) is... _____

MORNING THOUGHTS AND INSPIRATIONS

My biggest frog to eat today...
_____

ACTION STEPS FOR TODAY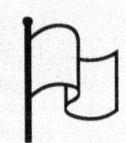

High Priority
1. _____
2. _____
3. _____

Medium Priority
1. _____
2. _____
3. _____

Low Priority
_____
_____
_____
_____
_____
_____

In which area(s) do I want to improve the most today?

Mental Health

Spiritual Health

Career Health

Physical Health

Social Health

Family Health

Financial Health

Weekly Goal Focus:

DAILY REVIEW
DAY 16

Today I am grateful for...

_____
_____
_____
_____
_____
_____
_____
_____

How was my day? Did I feel good about my performance? What did I learn? Did I have a new insight? What would I do differently?

_____
_____
_____
_____
_____
_____
_____
_____

NOTES AND REFLECTIONS FROM TODAY

What was my energy level today? (lowest to highest) 1 2 3 4 5 6 7 8 9 10

If not a "10", what will I do tomorrow to make it closer to a "10"? _____

I ate my frog today: Yes   No

What Time? _____

I did my new habit: Yes   No

What Time? _____

FOR TOMORROW

_____
_____
_____
_____

"Do not wait; the time will never be 'just right.' Start where you stand, and work with whatever tools you may have at your command, and better tools will be found as you go along."

Napoleon Hill

DAILY PREVIEW
DAY 17

M T W T F S S

Date: _____

MY PRIMARY OBJECTIVE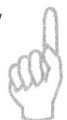

[   ]

The most important thing I can do today to take me a step closer to my Primary Objective is _____ .

The most important thing I can do today to take me a step closer to my Primary Objective is _____ .

The most important thing I can do today to take me a step closer to my Primary Objective is _____ .

The most important thing I can do today to take me a step closer to my Primary Objective is _____ .

My new habit I'm developing (eliminating) is… _____

MORNING THOUGHTS AND INSPIRATIONS

My biggest frog to eat today...
_____

ACTION STEPS FOR TODAY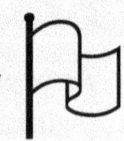

High Priority
1. _____
2. _____
3. _____

Medium Priority
1. _____
2. _____
3. _____

Low Priority
_____
_____
_____
_____
_____
_____

In which area(s) do I want to improve the most today?

Mental Health

Spiritual Health

Career Health

Physical Health

Social Health

Family Health

Financial Health

Weekly Goal Focus:

DAILY REVIEW
DAY 17

Today I am grateful for...

_____
_____
_____
_____
_____
_____
_____
_____

How was my day? Did I feel good about my performance? What did I learn? Did I have a new insight? What would I do differently?

_____
_____
_____
_____
_____
_____
_____

NOTES AND REFLECTIONS FROM TODAY

What was my energy level today? (lowest to highest)   1 2 3 4 5 6 7 8 9 10

If not a "10", what will I do tomorrow to make it closer to a "10"? _____

I ate my frog today: Yes   No

What Time? _____

I did my new habit: Yes   No

What Time? _____

FOR TOMORROW

_____
_____
_____
_____

"Act, look, feel successful, conduct yourself accordingly, and you will be amazed at the positive results."

William James

Life Alchemy 1.0   43

DAILY PREVIEW
DAY 18

M T W T F S S

Date: _____

MY PRIMARY OBJECTIVE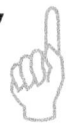

_____

The most important thing I can do today to take me a step closer to my Primary Objective is _____.

The most important thing I can do today to take me a step closer to my Primary Objective is _____.

The most important thing I can do today to take me a step closer to my Primary Objective is _____.

The most important thing I can do today to take me a step closer to my Primary Objective is _____.

My new habit I'm developing (eliminating) is... _____

MORNING THOUGHTS AND INSPIRATIONS

My biggest frog to eat today...
_____

ACTION STEPS FOR TODAY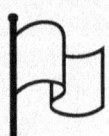

High Priority
1. _____
2. _____
3. _____

Medium Priority
1. _____
2. _____
3. _____

Low Priority
_____
_____
_____
_____
_____
_____

In which area(s) do I want to improve the most today?

Mental Health

Spiritual Health

Career Health

Physical Health

Social Health

Family Health

Financial Health

Weekly Goal Focus:

DAILY REVIEW
DAY 18

Today I am grateful for...

_____
_____
_____
_____
_____
_____
_____
_____

How was my day? Did I feel good about my performance? What did I learn? Did I have a new insight? What would I do differently?

_____
_____
_____
_____
_____
_____
_____

NOTES AND REFLECTIONS FROM TODAY

What was my energy level today? (lowest to highest) 1 2 3 4 5 6 7 8 9 10

If not a "10", what will I do tomorrow to make it closer to a "10"? _____

I ate my frog today: Yes   No

What Time? _____

I did my new habit: Yes   No

What Time? _____

FOR TOMORROW

_____
_____
_____
_____

"Success depends upon previous preparation, and without such preparation there is sure to be failure."
    Confucius

Life Alchemy 1.0

DAILY PREVIEW
DAY 19

M T W T F S S

Date: _____

MY PRIMARY OBJECTIVE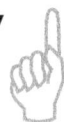

[   ]

The most important thing I can do today to take me a step closer to my Primary Objective is _____.

The most important thing I can do today to take me a step closer to my Primary Objective is _____.

The most important thing I can do today to take me a step closer to my Primary Objective is _____.

The most important thing I can do today to take me a step closer to my Primary Objective is _____.

My new habit I'm developing (eliminating) is... _____

MORNING THOUGHTS AND INSPIRATIONS

My biggest frog to eat today...
_____

ACTION STEPS FOR TODAY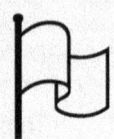

High Priority
1. _____
2. _____
3. _____

Medium Priority
1. _____
2. _____
3. _____

Low Priority
_____
_____
_____
_____
_____
_____

In which area(s) do I want to improve the most today?

Mental Health

Spiritual Health

Career Health

Physical Health

Social Health

Family Health

Financial Health

Weekly Goal Focus:

DAILY REVIEW
DAY 19

Today I am grateful for...

_____
_____
_____
_____
_____
_____
_____
_____

How was my day? Did I feel good about my performance? What did I learn? Did I have a new insight? What would I do differently?

_____
_____
_____
_____
_____
_____
_____

NOTES AND REFLECTIONS FROM TODAY

What was my energy level today? (lowest to highest) 1 2 3 4 5 6 7 8 9 10

If not a "10", what will I do tomorrow to make it closer to a "10"? _____

I ate my frog today: Yes   No

What Time? _____

I did my new habit: Yes   No

What Time? _____

FOR TOMORROW

_____
_____
_____
_____

"He has achieved success who has worked well, laughed often, and loved much."

— Elbert Hubbard

Life Alchemy 1.0

DAILY PREVIEW
DAY 20

M T W T F S S
Date: _____

MY PRIMARY OBJECTIVE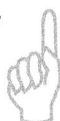

[_____]

The most important thing I can do today to take me a step closer to my Primary Objective is _____.

The most important thing I can do today to take me a step closer to my Primary Objective is _____.

The most important thing I can do today to take me a step closer to my Primary Objective is _____.

The most important thing I can do today to take me a step closer to my Primary Objective is _____.

My new habit I'm developing (eliminating) is… _____

MORNING THOUGHTS AND INSPIRATIONS

[   ]

My biggest frog to eat today…
_____

ACTION STEPS FOR TODAY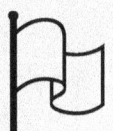

High Priority
1. _____
2. _____
3. _____

Medium Priority
1. _____
2. _____
3. _____

Low Priority
_____
_____
_____
_____
_____
_____

In which area(s) do I want to improve the most today?

Mental Health
Spiritual Health
Career Health
Physical Health
Social Health
Family Health
Financial Health

Weekly Goal Focus:

DAILY REVIEW
DAY 20

Today I am grateful for...

_____
_____
_____
_____
_____
_____
_____
_____

How was my day? Did I feel good about my performance? What did I learn? Did I have a new insight? What would I do differently?

_____
_____
_____
_____
_____
_____
_____
_____

NOTES AND REFLECTIONS FROM TODAY

What was my energy level today? (lowest to highest) 1 2 3 4 5 6 7 8 9 10

If not a "10", what will I do tomorrow to make it closer to a "10"? _____

I ate my frog today: Yes   No

What Time? _____

I did my new habit: Yes   No

What Time? _____

"Success isn't a result of spontaneous combustion. You must set yourself on fire."

Arnold H. Glasow

FOR TOMORROW

_____
_____
_____
_____

Life Alchemy 1.0

DAILY PREVIEW
DAY 21

M T W T F S S

Date: _____

MY PRIMARY OBJECTIVE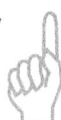

[_____]

The most important thing I can do today to take me a step closer to my Primary Objective is _____.

The most important thing I can do today to take me a step closer to my Primary Objective is _____.

The most important thing I can do today to take me a step closer to my Primary Objective is _____.

The most important thing I can do today to take me a step closer to my Primary Objective is _____.

My new habit I'm developing (eliminating) is... _____

MORNING THOUGHTS AND INSPIRATIONS

My biggest frog to eat today...
_____

ACTION STEPS FOR TODAY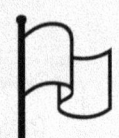

High Priority
1. _____
2. _____
3. _____

Medium Priority
1. _____
2. _____
3. _____

Low Priority
_____
_____
_____
_____
_____
_____

In which area(s) do I want to improve the most today?

Mental Health

Spiritual Health

Career Health

Physical Health

Social Health

Family Health

Financial Health

Weekly Goal Focus:

DAILY REVIEW
DAY 21

Today I am grateful for...

_____
_____
_____
_____
_____
_____
_____
_____

How was my day? Did I feel good about my performance? What did I learn? Did I have a new insight? What would I do differently?

_____
_____
_____
_____
_____
_____
_____
_____

NOTES AND REFLECTIONS FROM TODAY

What was my energy level today? (lowest to highest)   1 2 3 4 5 6 7 8 9 10

If not a "10", what will I do tomorrow to make it closer to a "10"? _____

I ate my frog today: Yes   No

What Time? _____

I did my new habit: Yes   No

What Time? _____

FOR TOMORROW

_____
_____
_____
_____

"There is only one success – to be able to spend your life in your own way."
Christopher Morley

Life Alchemy 1.0

WEEKLY CHECK-INS
WEEK 3

The Purpose of the Weekly Check-In is to...

1) Check-in with your progress throughout the week.

2) Re-focus for the upcoming week.

3) Get inspired for the future.

THE CHECK-IN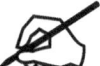

What have I accomplished since last week? What were the two most important things that I learned this week? Is there anything that I would have done differently? If so, what?

_____
_____
_____
_____
_____

What are my wins or victories since last week?

_____
_____
_____

What's the highlight (or low-light) of my week?

_____
_____
_____

What am I thankful for this week?

_____
_____
_____

The place I feel stuck is

_____
_____
_____

In which area(s) did I grow the most last week?

Mental Health

Spiritual Health

Career Health

Physical Health

Social Health

Family Health

Financial Health

What was my average energy level for the week?

1 2 3 4 5 6 7 8 9 10

What number do I want it to be next week?

1 2 3 4 5 6 7 8 9 10

How often did you eat your frog?

1 2 3 4 5 6 7

On a 1 - 10 scale, 1 being low and 10 being high, how grateful have I been feeling this last week?

1 2 3 4 5 6 7 8 9 10

How did I do with my new habit building/eliminating?

_____
_____
_____

RE-FOCUS WEEK 3

Every week, we will be re-focusing on our future life. So, take a moment and fill this in again. There will be a few questions after you finish.

If there were no rules, and I could not fail, what would my life be like?

Describe your future life in detail and in writing...

_____
_____
_____
_____
_____
_____
_____

When you wrote this out again, how did you feel? Were you excited? Were you bored? Did your vision evolve? Was it different than before? Was there more detail or less? Did you even do this exercise? If not, how come?

_____
_____
_____

Look through your future life. Now, fill in the blank...

If I only accomplish _____ next week, my future life would surely come to be.

This is your Primary Objective for the next week.

Take a moment and fill in the days of the week for the next week.

Go on to Day 22 and be amazing!

Life Alchemy 1.0

DAILY PREVIEW
DAY 22

M T W T F S S

Date: _____

MY PRIMARY OBJECTIVE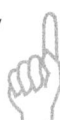

The most important thing I can do today to take me a step closer to my Primary Objective is _____.

The most important thing I can do today to take me a step closer to my Primary Objective is _____.

The most important thing I can do today to take me a step closer to my Primary Objective is _____.

The most important thing I can do today to take me a step closer to my Primary Objective is _____.

My new habit I'm developing (eliminating) is... _____

MORNING THOUGHTS AND INSPIRATIONS

My biggest frog to eat today...
_____

ACTION STEPS FOR TODAY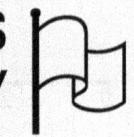

High Priority
1. _____
2. _____
3. _____

Medium Priority
1. _____
2. _____
3. _____

Low Priority
_____
_____
_____
_____
_____
_____

In which area(s) do I want to improve the most today?

Mental Health

Spiritual Health

Career Health

Physical Health

Social Health

Family Health

Financial Health

Weekly Goal Focus:

DAILY REVIEW
DAY 22

Today I am grateful for...

_____
_____
_____
_____
_____
_____
_____

How was my day? Did I feel good about my performance? What did I learn? Did I have a new insight? What would I do differently?

_____
_____
_____
_____
_____
_____
_____

NOTES AND REFLECTIONS FROM TODAY

What was my energy level today? (lowest to highest)   1 2 3 4 5 6 7 8 9 10

If not a "10", what will I do tomorrow to make it closer to a "10"? _____

I ate my frog today: Yes   No

What Time? _____

I did my new habit: Yes   No

What Time? _____

FOR TOMORROW

_____
_____
_____
_____

"Nothing succeeds like success."
Alexandre Dumas

Life Alchemy 1.0

DAILY PREVIEW
DAY 23

M T W T F S S

Date: _____

MY PRIMARY OBJECTIVE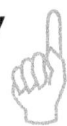

The most important thing I can do today to take me a step closer to my Primary Objective is _____.

The most important thing I can do today to take me a step closer to my Primary Objective is _____.

The most important thing I can do today to take me a step closer to my Primary Objective is _____.

The most important thing I can do today to take me a step closer to my Primary Objective is _____.

My new habit I'm developing (eliminating) is... _____

MORNING THOUGHTS AND INSPIRATIONS

My biggest frog to eat today...
_____

ACTION STEPS FOR TODAY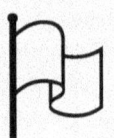

High Priority
1. _____
2. _____
3. _____

Medium Priority
1. _____
2. _____
3. _____

Low Priority
_____
_____
_____
_____
_____
_____

In which area(s) do I want to improve the most today?

Mental Health

Spiritual Health

Career Health

Physical Health

Social Health

Family Health

Financial Health

Weekly Goal Focus:

DAILY REVIEW
DAY 23

Today I am grateful for...

_____
_____
_____
_____
_____
_____
_____
_____

How was my day? Did I feel good about my performance? What did I learn? Did I have a new insight? What would I do differently?

_____
_____
_____
_____
_____
_____
_____
_____

NOTES AND REFLECTIONS FROM TODAY

What was my energy level today? (lowest to highest) 1 2 3 4 5 6 7 8 9 10

If not a "10", what will I do tomorrow to make it closer to a "10"? _____

I ate my frog today: Yes   No

I did my new habit: Yes   No

What Time? _____

What Time? _____

FOR TOMORROW

_____
_____
_____
_____

"To live a creative life, we must lose our fear of being wrong."

Anonymous

Life Alchemy 1.0

DAILY PREVIEW
DAY 24

M T W T F S S

Date: _____

MY PRIMARY OBJECTIVE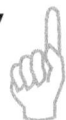

_____

The most important thing I can do today to take me a step closer to my Primary Objective is _____.

The most important thing I can do today to take me a step closer to my Primary Objective is _____.

The most important thing I can do today to take me a step closer to my Primary Objective is _____.

The most important thing I can do today to take me a step closer to my Primary Objective is _____.

My new habit I'm developing (eliminating) is... _____

MORNING THOUGHTS AND INSPIRATIONS

My biggest frog to eat today...
_____

ACTION STEPS FOR TODAY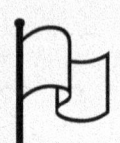

High Priority
1. _____
2. _____
3. _____

Medium Priority
1. _____
2. _____
3. _____

Low Priority
_____
_____
_____
_____
_____
_____

In which area(s) do I want to improve the most today?

Mental Health

Spiritual Health

Career Health

Physical Health

Social Health

Family Health

Financial Health

Weekly Goal Focus:

DAILY REVIEW
DAY 24

Today I am grateful for...

How was my day? Did I feel good about my performance? What did I learn? Did I have a new insight? What would I do differently?

NOTES AND REFLECTIONS FROM TODAY

What was my energy level today? (lowest to highest) 1 2 3 4 5 6 7 8 9 10

If not a "10", what will I do tomorrow to make it closer to a "10"? _____

I ate my frog today: Yes   No

I did my new habit: Yes   No

What Time? _____

What Time? _____

FOR TOMORROW

"All our dreams can come true if we have the courage to pursue them."
— *Walt Disney*

Life Alchemy 1.0

DAILY PREVIEW
DAY 25

M T W T F S S

Date: _____

MY PRIMARY OBJECTIVE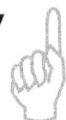

_____

The most important thing I can do today to take me a step closer to my Primary Objective is _____.

The most important thing I can do today to take me a step closer to my Primary Objective is _____.

The most important thing I can do today to take me a step closer to my Primary Objective is _____.

The most important thing I can do today to take me a step closer to my Primary Objective is _____.

My new habit I'm developing (eliminating) is... _____

MORNING THOUGHTS AND INSPIRATIONS

My biggest frog to eat today...
_____

ACTION STEPS FOR TODAY

High Priority
1. _____
2. _____
3. _____

Medium Priority
1. _____
2. _____
3. _____

Low Priority
_____
_____
_____
_____
_____
_____

In which area(s) do I want to improve the most today?

Mental Health

Spiritual Health

Career Health

Physical Health

Social Health

Family Health

Financial Health

Weekly Goal Focus:

DAILY REVIEW
DAY 25

Today I am grateful for...

_____
_____
_____
_____
_____
_____
_____
_____

How was my day? Did I feel good about my performance? What did I learn? Did I have a new insight? What would I do differently?

_____
_____
_____
_____
_____
_____
_____
_____

NOTES AND REFLECTIONS FROM TODAY

What was my energy level today? (lowest to highest) 1 2 3 4 5 6 7 8 9 10

If not a "10", what will I do tomorrow to make it closer to a "10"? _____

I ate my frog today: Yes   No

What Time? _____

I did my new habit: Yes   No

What Time? _____

FOR TOMORROW

_____
_____
_____
_____
_____

"Opportunities don't happen, you create them."

Chris Grosser

Life Alchemy 1.0

DAILY PREVIEW
DAY 26

M T W T F S S

Date: _____

MY PRIMARY OBJECTIVE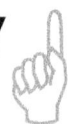

The most important thing I can do today to take me a step closer to my Primary Objective is _____ .

The most important thing I can do today to take me a step closer to my Primary Objective is _____ .

The most important thing I can do today to take me a step closer to my Primary Objective is _____ .

The most important thing I can do today to take me a step closer to my Primary Objective is _____ .

My new habit I'm developing (eliminating) is... _____

MORNING THOUGHTS AND INSPIRATIONS

My biggest frog to eat today...
_____

ACTION STEPS FOR TODAY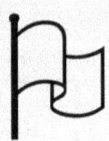

High Priority
1. _____
2. _____
3. _____

Medium Priority
1. _____
2. _____
3. _____

Low Priority
_____
_____
_____
_____
_____
_____

In which area(s) do I want to improve the most today?

Mental Health

Spiritual Health

Career Health

Physical Health

Social Health

Family Health

Financial Health

Weekly Goal Focus:

DAILY REVIEW
DAY 26

Today I am grateful for...

_____
_____
_____
_____
_____
_____
_____
_____

How was my day? Did I feel good about my performance? What did I learn? Did I have a new insight? What would I do differently?

_____
_____
_____
_____
_____
_____
_____
_____

NOTES AND REFLECTIONS FROM TODAY

What was my energy level today? (lowest to highest)   1 2 3 4 5 6 7 8 9 10

If not a "10", what will I do tomorrow to make it closer to a "10"? _____

I ate my frog today: Yes   No

I did my new habit: Yes   No

What Time? _____

What Time? _____

FOR TOMORROW

_____
_____
_____
_____

"No one can make you feel inferior without your consent."

Eleanor Roosevelt

DAILY PREVIEW
DAY 27

M T W T F S S
Date: _____

MY PRIMARY OBJECTIVE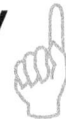

[   ]

The most important thing I can do today to take me a step closer to my Primary Objective is _____.

The most important thing I can do today to take me a step closer to my Primary Objective is _____.

The most important thing I can do today to take me a step closer to my Primary Objective is _____.

The most important thing I can do today to take me a step closer to my Primary Objective is _____.

My new habit I'm developing (eliminating) is... _____

MORNING THOUGHTS AND INSPIRATIONS

My biggest frog to eat today...
_____

ACTION STEPS FOR TODAY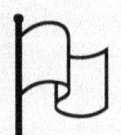

High Priority
1. _____
2. _____
3. _____

Medium Priority
1. _____
2. _____
3. _____

Low Priority
_____
_____
_____
_____
_____
_____

In which area(s) do I want to improve the most today?

Mental Health
Spiritual Health
Career Health
Physical Health
Social Health
Family Health
Financial Health

Weekly Goal Focus:

DAILY REVIEW
DAY 27

Today I am grateful for...

How was my day? Did I feel good about my performance? What did I learn? Did I have a new insight? What would I do differently?

NOTES AND REFLECTIONS FROM TODAY

What was my energy level today? (lowest to highest) 1 2 3 4 5 6 7 8 9 10

If not a "10", what will I do tomorrow to make it closer to a "10"? _____

I ate my frog today: Yes   No   I did my new habit: Yes   No

What Time? _____   What Time? _____

FOR TOMORROW

"The ones who are crazy enough to think they can change the world, are the ones that do."

Anonymous

Life Alchemy 1.0

DAILY PREVIEW
DAY 28

M T W T F S S

Date: _____

MY PRIMARY OBJECTIVE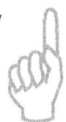

[_____]

The most important thing I can do today to take me a step closer to my Primary Objective is _____ .

The most important thing I can do today to take me a step closer to my Primary Objective is _____ .

The most important thing I can do today to take me a step closer to my Primary Objective is _____ .

The most important thing I can do today to take me a step closer to my Primary Objective is _____ .

My new habit I'm developing (eliminating) is... _____

MORNING THOUGHTS AND INSPIRATIONS

My biggest frog to eat today...
_____

ACTION STEPS FOR TODAY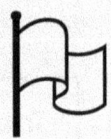

High Priority
1. _____
2. _____
3. _____

Medium Priority
1. _____
2. _____
3. _____

Low Priority
_____
_____
_____
_____
_____

In which area(s) do I want to improve the most today?

Mental Health

Spiritual Health

Career Health

Physical Health

Social Health

Family Health

Financial Health

DAILY REVIEW
DAY 28

Weekly Goal Focus:

Today I am grateful for...
_____
_____
_____
_____
_____
_____
_____
_____

How was my day? Did I feel good about my performance? What did I learn? Did I have a new insight? What would I do differently?
_____
_____
_____
_____
_____
_____
_____
_____

NOTES AND REFLECTIONS FROM TODAY

What was my energy level today? (lowest to highest) 1 2 3 4 5 6 7 8 9 10

If not a "10", what will I do tomorrow to make it closer to a "10"? _____

I ate my frog today: Yes   No

I did my new habit: Yes   No

What Time? _____

What Time? _____

FOR TOMORROW
_____
_____
_____
_____

"What seems to us as bitter trials are often blessings in disguise."

— Oscar Wilde

Life Alchemy 1.0

WEEKLY CHECK-INS
WEEK 4

The Purpose of the Weekly Check-In is to...

1) Check-in with your progress throughout the week.

2) Re-focus for the upcoming week.

3) Get inspired for the future.

THE CHECK-IN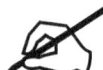

What have I accomplished since last week? What were the two most important things that I learned this week? Is there anything that I would have done differently? If so, what?

_____
_____
_____
_____
_____

What are my wins or victories since last week?

_____
_____
_____

What's the highlight (or low-light) of my week?

_____
_____
_____

What am I thankful for this week?

_____
_____
_____
_____

The place I feel stuck is

_____
_____
_____

In which area(s) did I grow the most last week?

Mental Health

Spiritual Health

Career Health

Physical Health

Social Health

Family Health

Financial Health

What was my average energy level for the week?

1 2 3 4 5 6 7 8 9 10

What number do I want it to be next week?

1 2 3 4 5 6 7 8 9 10

How often did you eat your frog?

1 2 3 4 5 6 7

On a 1 - 10 scale, 1 being low and 10 being high, how grateful have I been feeling this last week?

1 2 3 4 5 6 7 8 9 10

How did I do with my new habit building/eliminating?

_____
_____
_____

RE-FOCUS WEEK 4

Every week, we will be re-focusing on our future life. So, take a moment and fill this in again. There will be a few questions after you finish.

If there were no rules, and I could not fail, what would my life be like?

Describe your future life in detail and in writing...

_____
_____
_____
_____
_____
_____
_____

When you wrote this out again, how did you feel? Were you excited? Were you bored? Did your vision evolve? Was it different than before? Was there more detail or less? Did you even do this exercise? If not, how come?

_____
_____
_____

Look through your future life. Now, fill in the blank...

If I only accomplish _____ next week, my future life would surely come to be.

This is your Primary Objective for the next week.

Take a moment and fill in the days of the week for the next week.

Go on to Day 29 and be amazing!

Life Alchemy 1.0

DAILY PREVIEW
DAY 29

M T W T F S S

Date: _____

MY PRIMARY OBJECTIVE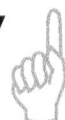

[_____]

The most important thing I can do today to take me a step closer to my Primary Objective is _____.

The most important thing I can do today to take me a step closer to my Primary Objective is _____.

The most important thing I can do today to take me a step closer to my Primary Objective is _____.

The most important thing I can do today to take me a step closer to my Primary Objective is _____.

My new habit I'm developing (eliminating) is... _____

MORNING THOUGHTS AND INSPIRATIONS

My biggest frog to eat today...
_____

ACTION STEPS FOR TODAY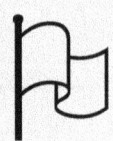

High Priority
1. _____
2. _____
3. _____

Medium Priority
1. _____
2. _____
3. _____

Low Priority
_____
_____
_____
_____
_____
_____

In which area(s) do I want to improve the most today?

Mental Health

Spiritual Health

Career Health

Physical Health

Social Health

Family Health

Financial Health

Weekly Goal Focus:

DAILY REVIEW
DAY 29

Today I am grateful for...

_____
_____
_____
_____
_____
_____
_____

How was my day? Did I feel good about my performance? What did I learn? Did I have a new insight? What would I do differently?

_____
_____
_____
_____
_____
_____
_____

NOTES AND REFLECTIONS FROM TODAY

What was my energy level today? (lowest to highest)   1 2 3 4 5 6 7 8 9 10

If not a "10", what will I do tomorrow to make it closer to a "10"? _____

I ate my frog today: Yes   No

I did my new habit: Yes   No

What Time? _____

What Time? _____

FOR TOMORROW

_____
_____
_____
_____

*"The meaning of life is to find your gift.
The purpose of life is to give it away."*
        — Anonymous

Life Alchemy 1.0

DAILY PREVIEW
DAY 30

M T W T F S S

Date: _____

MY PRIMARY OBJECTIVE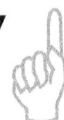

[_____]

The most important thing I can do today to take me a step closer to my Primary Objective is _____.

The most important thing I can do today to take me a step closer to my Primary Objective is _____.

The most important thing I can do today to take me a step closer to my Primary Objective is _____.

The most important thing I can do today to take me a step closer to my Primary Objective is _____.

My new habit I'm developing (eliminating) is... _____

MORNING THOUGHTS AND INSPIRATIONS

My biggest frog to eat today...
_____

ACTION STEPS FOR TODAY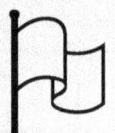

High Priority
1. _____
2. _____
3. _____

Medium Priority
1. _____
2. _____
3. _____

Low Priority
_____
_____
_____
_____
_____
_____

In which area(s) do I want to improve the most today?

Mental Health

Spiritual Health

Career Health

Physical Health

Social Health

Family Health

Financial Health

Weekly Goal Focus:

DAILY REVIEW
DAY 30

Today I am grateful for...

_____
_____
_____
_____
_____
_____
_____
_____

How was my day? Did I feel good about my performance? What did I learn? Did I have a new insight? What would I do differently?

_____
_____
_____
_____
_____
_____
_____

NOTES AND REFLECTIONS FROM TODAY

What was my energy level today? (lowest to highest)   1 2 3 4 5 6 7 8 9 10

If not a "10", what will I do tomorrow to make it closer to a "10"? _____

I ate my frog today: Yes   No

What Time? _____

I did my new habit: Yes   No

What Time? _____

FOR TOMORROW

_____
_____
_____
_____

"The distance between insanity and genius is measured only by success."
Bruce Feirstein

Life Alchemy 1.0

DAILY PREVIEW
DAY 31

M T W T F S S

Date: _____

MY PRIMARY OBJECTIVE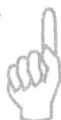

The most important thing I can do today to take me a step closer to my Primary Objective is _____ .

The most important thing I can do today to take me a step closer to my Primary Objective is _____ .

The most important thing I can do today to take me a step closer to my Primary Objective is _____ .

The most important thing I can do today to take me a step closer to my Primary Objective is _____ .

My new habit I'm developing (eliminating) is... _____

MORNING THOUGHTS AND INSPIRATIONS

My biggest frog to eat today...
_____

ACTION STEPS FOR TODAY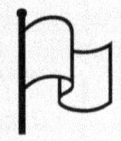

High Priority
1. _____
2. _____
3. _____

Medium Priority
1. _____
2. _____
3. _____

Low Priority
_____
_____
_____
_____
_____
_____

In which area(s) do I want to improve the most today?

Mental Health

Spiritual Health

Career Health

Physical Health

Social Health

Family Health

Financial Health

Weekly Goal Focus:

DAILY REVIEW
DAY 31

Today I am grateful for...

How was my day? Did I feel good about my performance? What did I learn? Did I have a new insight? What would I do differently?

NOTES AND REFLECTIONS FROM TODAY

What was my energy level today? (lowest to highest) 1 2 3 4 5 6 7 8 9 10

If not a "10", what will I do tomorrow to make it closer to a "10"? _____

I ate my frog today: Yes   No

I did my new habit: Yes   No

What Time? _____

What Time? _____

FOR TOMORROW

"Don't be afraid to give up the good to go for the great."

— John D. Rockefeller

Life Alchemy 1.0

DAILY PREVIEW
DAY 32

M T W T F S S

Date: _____

My biggest frog to eat today...
_____

ACTION STEPS FOR TODAY

MY PRIMARY OBJECTIVE 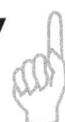 _____

The most important thing I can do today to take me a step closer to my Primary Objective is _____.

The most important thing I can do today to take me a step closer to my Primary Objective is _____.

The most important thing I can do today to take me a step closer to my Primary Objective is _____.

The most important thing I can do today to take me a step closer to my Primary Objective is _____.

My new habit I'm developing (eliminating) is... _____

High Priority
1. _____
2. _____
3. _____

Medium Priority
1. _____
2. _____
3. _____

Low Priority
_____
_____
_____
_____
_____
_____

MORNING THOUGHTS AND INSPIRATIONS

In which area(s) do I want to improve the most today?

Mental Health

Spiritual Health

Career Health

Physical Health

Social Health

Family Health

Financial Health

Weekly Goal Focus:

DAILY REVIEW
DAY 32

Today I am grateful for...

How was my day? Did I feel good about my performance? What did I learn? Did I have a new insight? What would I do differently?

NOTES AND REFLECTIONS FROM TODAY

What was my energy level today? (lowest to highest) 1 2 3 4 5 6 7 8 9 10

If not a "10", what will I do tomorrow to make it closer to a "10"? _____

I ate my frog today: Yes   No

I did my new habit: Yes   No

What Time? _____

What Time? _____

FOR TOMORROW

"Do one thing every day that scares you."

Anonymous

Life Alchemy 1.0   77

DAILY PREVIEW
DAY 33

M T W T F S S

Date: _____

MY PRIMARY OBJECTIVE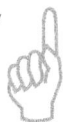

[_____]

The most important thing I can do today to take me a step closer to my Primary Objective is _____.

The most important thing I can do today to take me a step closer to my Primary Objective is _____.

The most important thing I can do today to take me a step closer to my Primary Objective is _____.

The most important thing I can do today to take me a step closer to my Primary Objective is _____.

My new habit I'm developing (eliminating) is... _____

MORNING THOUGHTS AND INSPIRATIONS

My biggest frog to eat today...
_____

ACTION STEPS FOR TODAY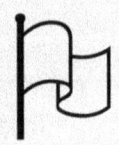

High Priority
1. _____
2. _____
3. _____

Medium Priority
1. _____
2. _____
3. _____

Low Priority
_____
_____
_____
_____
_____
_____

In which area(s) do I want to improve the most today?

Mental Health

Spiritual Health

Career Health

Physical Health

Social Health

Family Health

Financial Health

Weekly Goal Focus:

DAILY REVIEW
DAY 33

Today I am grateful for...

How was my day? Did I feel good about my performance? What did I learn? Did I have a new insight? What would I do differently?

NOTES AND REFLECTIONS FROM TODAY

What was my energy level today? (lowest to highest) 1 2 3 4 5 6 7 8 9 10

If not a "10", what will I do tomorrow to make it closer to a "10"? _____

I ate my frog today: Yes   No

I did my new habit: Yes   No

What Time? _____

What Time? _____

FOR TOMORROW

"Life is not about finding yourself. Life is about creating yourself."

Lolly Daskal

Life Alchemy 1.0

DAILY PREVIEW
DAY 34

M T W T F S S

Date: _____

MY PRIMARY OBJECTIVE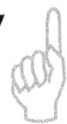

 _____

The most important thing I can do today to take me a step closer to my Primary Objective is _____.

The most important thing I can do today to take me a step closer to my Primary Objective is _____.

The most important thing I can do today to take me a step closer to my Primary Objective is _____.

The most important thing I can do today to take me a step closer to my Primary Objective is _____.

My new habit I'm developing (eliminating) is... _____

MORNING THOUGHTS AND INSPIRATIONS

My biggest frog to eat today...
_____

ACTION STEPS FOR TODAY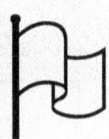

High Priority
1. _____
2. _____
3. _____

Medium Priority
1. _____
2. _____
3. _____

Low Priority
_____
_____
_____
_____
_____
_____

In which area(s) do I want to improve the most today?

Mental Health

Spiritual Health

Career Health

Physical Health

Social Health

Family Health

Financial Health

Weekly Goal Focus:

DAILY REVIEW
DAY 34

Today I am grateful for...

_____
_____
_____
_____
_____
_____
_____
_____

How was my day? Did I feel good about my performance? What did I learn? Did I have a new insight? What would I do differently?

_____
_____
_____
_____
_____
_____
_____
_____

NOTES AND REFLECTIONS FROM TODAY

What was my energy level today? (lowest to highest)   1 2 3 4 5 6 7 8 9 10

If not a "10", what will I do tomorrow to make it closer to a "10"? _____

I ate my frog today: Yes   No

What Time? _____

I did my new habit: Yes   No

What Time? _____

FOR TOMORROW

_____
_____
_____
_____

"You can do anything, but not everything."

Anonymous

Life Alchemy 1.0

DAILY PREVIEW
DAY 35

M T W T F S S

Date: _____

MY PRIMARY OBJECTIVE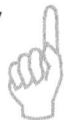

[   ]

The most important thing I can do today to take me a step closer to my Primary Objective is _____.

The most important thing I can do today to take me a step closer to my Primary Objective is _____.

The most important thing I can do today to take me a step closer to my Primary Objective is _____.

The most important thing I can do today to take me a step closer to my Primary Objective is _____.

My new habit I'm developing (eliminating) is... _____

MORNING THOUGHTS AND INSPIRATIONS

My biggest frog to eat today...
_____

ACTION STEPS FOR TODAY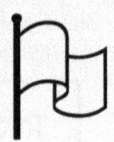

High Priority
1. _____
2. _____
3. _____

Medium Priority
1. _____
2. _____
3. _____

Low Priority
_____
_____
_____
_____
_____
_____

In which area(s) do I want to improve the most today?

Mental Health

Spiritual Health

Career Health

Physical Health

Social Health

Family Health

Financial Health

Weekly Goal Focus:

DAILY REVIEW
DAY 35

Today I am grateful for...

_____
_____
_____
_____
_____
_____
_____
_____

How was my day? Did I feel good about my performance? What did I learn? Did I have a new insight? What would I do differently?

_____
_____
_____
_____
_____
_____
_____
_____

NOTES AND REFLECTIONS FROM TODAY

What was my energy level today? (lowest to highest)   1 2 3 4 5 6 7 8 9 10

If not a "10", what will I do tomorrow to make it closer to a "10"? _____

I ate my frog today: Yes   No

What Time? _____

I did my new habit: Yes   No

What Time? _____

"I find that the harder I work, the more luck I seem to have."

Thomas Jefferson

FOR TOMORROW

_____
_____
_____
_____

Life Alchemy 1.0

WEEKLY CHECK-INS
WEEK 5

The Purpose of the Weekly Check-In is to...

1) Check-in with your progress throughout the week.

2) Re-focus for the upcoming week.

3) Get inspired for the future.

THE CHECK-IN

What have I accomplished since last week? What were the two most important things that I learned this week? Is there anything that I would have done differently? If so, what?

_____
_____
_____
_____

What are my wins or victories since last week?

_____
_____
_____

What's the highlight (or low-light) of my week?

_____
_____
_____

What am I thankful for this week?

_____
_____
_____

The place I feel stuck is

_____
_____
_____

In which area(s) did I grow the most last week?

Mental Health

Spiritual Health

Career Health

Physical Health

Social Health

Family Health

Financial Health

What was my average energy level for the week?

1 2 3 4 5 6 7 8 9 10

What number do I want it to be next week?

1 2 3 4 5 6 7 8 9 10

How often did you eat your frog?

1 2 3 4 5 6 7

On a 1 - 10 scale, 1 being low and 10 being high, how grateful have I been feeling this last week?

1 2 3 4 5 6 7 8 9 10

How did I do with my new habit building/eliminating?

_____
_____
_____

RE-FOCUS WEEK 5

Every week, we will be re-focusing on our future life. So, take a moment and fill this in again. There will be a few questions after you finish.

If there were no rules, and I could not fail, what would my life be like?

Describe your future life in detail and in writing...

_____
_____
_____
_____
_____
_____
_____

When you wrote this out again, how did you feel? Were you excited? Were you bored? Did your vision evolve? Was it different than before? Was there more detail or less? Did you even do this exercise? If not, how come?

_____
_____
_____

Look through your future life. Now, fill in the blank...

If I only accomplish _____ next week, my future life would surely come to be.

This is your Primary Objective for the next week.

Take a moment and fill in the days of the week for the next week.

Go on to Day 36 and be amazing!

Life Alchemy 1.0

DAILY PREVIEW
DAY 36

M T W T F S S

Date: _____

MY PRIMARY OBJECTIVE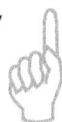

_____

The most important thing I can do today to take me a step closer to my Primary Objective is _____ .

The most important thing I can do today to take me a step closer to my Primary Objective is _____ .

The most important thing I can do today to take me a step closer to my Primary Objective is _____ .

The most important thing I can do today to take me a step closer to my Primary Objective is _____ .

My new habit I'm developing (eliminating) is... _____

MORNING THOUGHTS AND INSPIRATIONS

My biggest frog to eat today...
_____

ACTION STEPS FOR TODAY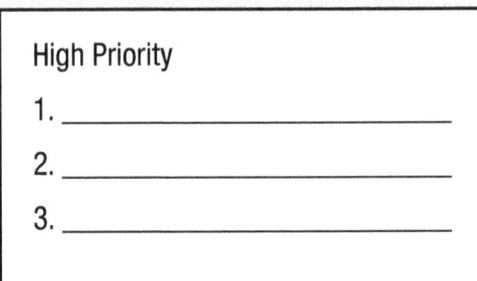

High Priority
1. _____
2. _____
3. _____

Medium Priority
1. _____
2. _____
3. _____

Low Priority
_____
_____
_____
_____
_____
_____

In which area(s) do I want to improve the most today?

Mental Health

Spiritual Health

Career Health

Physical Health

Social Health

Family Health

Financial Health

Weekly Goal Focus:

DAILY REVIEW
DAY 36

Today I am grateful for...

How was my day? Did I feel good about my performance? What did I learn? Did I have a new insight? What would I do differently?

NOTES AND REFLECTIONS FROM TODAY

What was my energy level today? (lowest to highest)   1 2 3 4 5 6 7 8 9 10

If not a "10", what will I do tomorrow to make it closer to a "10"? _____

I ate my frog today: Yes   No

What Time? _____

I did my new habit: Yes   No

What Time? _____

FOR TOMORROW

"Success is the sum of small efforts, repeated day-in and day-out."
Robert Collier

Life Alchemy 1.0

DAILY PREVIEW
DAY 37

M T W T F S S

Date: _____

MY PRIMARY OBJECTIVE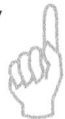

The most important thing I can do today to take me a step closer to my Primary Objective is _____ .

The most important thing I can do today to take me a step closer to my Primary Objective is _____ .

The most important thing I can do today to take me a step closer to my Primary Objective is _____ .

The most important thing I can do today to take me a step closer to my Primary Objective is _____ .

My new habit I'm developing (eliminating) is... _____

MORNING THOUGHTS AND INSPIRATIONS

My biggest frog to eat today...
_____

ACTION STEPS FOR TODAY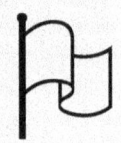

High Priority
1. _____
2. _____
3. _____

Medium Priority
1. _____
2. _____
3. _____

Low Priority
_____
_____
_____
_____
_____
_____

In which area(s) do I want to improve the most today?

Mental Health

Spiritual Health

Career Health

Physical Health

Social Health

Family Health

Financial Health

Weekly Goal Focus:

DAILY REVIEW
DAY 37

Today I am grateful for...

_____
_____
_____
_____
_____
_____
_____
_____

How was my day? Did I feel good about my performance? What did I learn? Did I have a new insight? What would I do differently?

_____
_____
_____
_____
_____
_____
_____

NOTES AND REFLECTIONS FROM TODAY

What was my energy level today? (lowest to highest) 1 2 3 4 5 6 7 8 9 10

If not a "10", what will I do tomorrow to make it closer to a "10"? _____

I ate my frog today: Yes   No

What Time? _____

I did my new habit: Yes   No

What Time? _____

FOR TOMORROW

_____
_____
_____
_____

"All progress takes place outside the comfort zone."

Michael John Bobak

Life Alchemy 1.0

DAILY PREVIEW
DAY 38

M T W T F S S

Date: _____

MY PRIMARY OBJECTIVE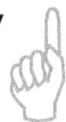

The most important thing I can do today to take me a step closer to my Primary Objective is _____.

The most important thing I can do today to take me a step closer to my Primary Objective is _____.

The most important thing I can do today to take me a step closer to my Primary Objective is _____.

The most important thing I can do today to take me a step closer to my Primary Objective is _____.

My new habit I'm developing (eliminating) is... _____

MORNING THOUGHTS AND INSPIRATIONS

My biggest frog to eat today...
_____

ACTION STEPS FOR TODAY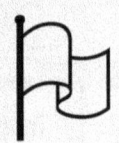

High Priority
1. _____
2. _____
3. _____

Medium Priority
1. _____
2. _____
3. _____

Low Priority
_____
_____
_____
_____
_____
_____

In which area(s) do I want to improve the most today?

Mental Health

Spiritual Health

Career Health

Physical Health

Social Health

Family Health

Financial Health

Weekly Goal Focus:

DAILY REVIEW
DAY 38

Today I am grateful for...

How was my day? Did I feel good about my performance? What did I learn? Did I have a new insight? What would I do differently?

NOTES AND REFLECTIONS FROM TODAY

What was my energy level today? (lowest to highest)   1 2 3 4 5 6 7 8 9 10

If not a "10", what will I do tomorrow to make it closer to a "10"? _____

I ate my frog today: Yes   No

I did my new habit: Yes   No

What Time? _____

What Time? _____

FOR TOMORROW

"The only place where success comes before work is in the dictionary."
Vidal Sassoon

Life Alchemy 1.0

DAILY PREVIEW
DAY 39

M T W T F S S

Date: _____

MY PRIMARY OBJECTIVE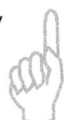

The most important thing I can do today to take me a step closer to my Primary Objective is _____.

The most important thing I can do today to take me a step closer to my Primary Objective is _____.

The most important thing I can do today to take me a step closer to my Primary Objective is _____.

The most important thing I can do today to take me a step closer to my Primary Objective is _____.

My new habit I'm developing (eliminating) is... _____

MORNING THOUGHTS AND INSPIRATIONS

My biggest frog to eat today...
_____

ACTION STEPS FOR TODAY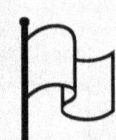

High Priority
1. _____
2. _____
3. _____

Medium Priority
1. _____
2. _____
3. _____

Low Priority
_____
_____
_____
_____
_____
_____

In which area(s) do I want to improve the most today?

Mental Health

Spiritual Health

Career Health

Physical Health

Social Health

Family Health

Financial Health

Weekly Goal Focus:

DAILY REVIEW
DAY 39

Today I am grateful for...

How was my day? Did I feel good about my performance? What did I learn? Did I have a new insight? What would I do differently?

NOTES AND REFLECTIONS FROM TODAY

What was my energy level today? (lowest to highest) 1 2 3 4 5 6 7 8 9 10

If not a "10", what will I do tomorrow to make it closer to a "10"? _____

I ate my frog today: Yes   No

I did my new habit: Yes   No

What Time? _____

What Time? _____

FOR TOMORROW

"Success is liking yourself, liking what you do, and liking how you do it."
Maya Angelou

Life Alchemy 1.0   93

DAILY PREVIEW
DAY 40

M T W T F S S

Date: _____

MY PRIMARY OBJECTIVE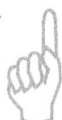

The most important thing I can do today to take me a step closer to my Primary Objective is _____.

The most important thing I can do today to take me a step closer to my Primary Objective is _____.

The most important thing I can do today to take me a step closer to my Primary Objective is _____.

The most important thing I can do today to take me a step closer to my Primary Objective is _____.

My new habit I'm developing (eliminating) is... _____

MORNING THOUGHTS AND INSPIRATIONS

My biggest frog to eat today...
_____

ACTION STEPS FOR TODAY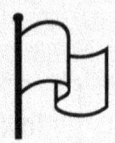

High Priority
1. _____
2. _____
3. _____

Medium Priority
1. _____
2. _____
3. _____

Low Priority
_____
_____
_____
_____
_____
_____

In which area(s) do I want to improve the most today?

Mental Health

Spiritual Health

Career Health

Physical Health

Social Health

Family Health

Financial Health

Weekly Goal Focus:

DAILY REVIEW
DAY 40

Today I am grateful for...

_____
_____
_____
_____
_____
_____
_____
_____

How was my day? Did I feel good about my performance? What did I learn? Did I have a new insight? What would I do differently?

_____
_____
_____
_____
_____
_____
_____
_____

NOTES AND REFLECTIONS FROM TODAY

What was my energy level today? (lowest to highest)   1 2 3 4 5 6 7 8 9 10

If not a "10", what will I do tomorrow to make it closer to a "10"? _____

I ate my frog today: Yes   No

I did my new habit: Yes   No

What Time? _____

What Time? _____

FOR TOMORROW

_____
_____
_____
_____

"When I dare to be powerful – to use my strength in the service of my vision, then it becomes less and less important whether I am afraid."

— Audre Lorde

Life Alchemy 1.0

DAILY PREVIEW
DAY 41

M T W T F S S

Date: _____

MY PRIMARY OBJECTIVE

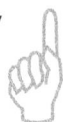

_____

The most important thing I can do today to take me a step closer to my Primary Objective is _____ .

The most important thing I can do today to take me a step closer to my Primary Objective is _____ .

The most important thing I can do today to take me a step closer to my Primary Objective is _____ .

The most important thing I can do today to take me a step closer to my Primary Objective is _____ .

My new habit I'm developing (eliminating) is... _____

MORNING THOUGHTS AND INSPIRATIONS

My biggest frog to eat today...
_____

ACTION STEPS FOR TODAY

High Priority
1. _____
2. _____
3. _____

Medium Priority
1. _____
2. _____
3. _____

Low Priority
_____
_____
_____
_____
_____
_____

In which area(s) do I want to improve the most today?

Mental Health

Spiritual Health

Career Health

Physical Health

Social Health

Family Health

Financial Health

Weekly Goal Focus:

DAILY REVIEW
DAY 41

Today I am grateful for...

How was my day? Did I feel good about my performance? What did I learn? Did I have a new insight? What would I do differently?

NOTES AND REFLECTIONS FROM TODAY

What was my energy level today? (lowest to highest) 1 2 3 4 5 6 7 8 9 10

If not a "10", what will I do tomorrow to make it closer to a "10"? _____

I ate my frog today: Yes   No

I did my new habit: Yes   No

What Time? _____

What Time? _____

FOR TOMORROW

"Success usually comes to those who are too busy to be looking for it."
— Henry David Thoreau

DAILY PREVIEW
DAY 42

M T W T F S S
Date: _____

MY PRIMARY OBJECTIVE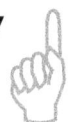

The most important thing I can do today to take me a step closer to my Primary Objective is _____.

The most important thing I can do today to take me a step closer to my Primary Objective is _____.

The most important thing I can do today to take me a step closer to my Primary Objective is _____.

The most important thing I can do today to take me a step closer to my Primary Objective is _____.

My new habit I'm developing (eliminating) is... _____

MORNING THOUGHTS AND INSPIRATIONS

My biggest frog to eat today...
_____

ACTION STEPS FOR TODAY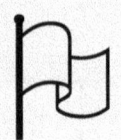

High Priority
1. _____
2. _____
3. _____

Medium Priority
1. _____
2. _____
3. _____

Low Priority
_____
_____
_____
_____
_____
_____

In which area(s) do I want to improve the most today?

Mental Health

Spiritual Health

Career Health

Physical Health

Social Health

Family Health

Financial Health

DAILY REVIEW
DAY 42

Weekly Goal Focus:

Today I am grateful for...

_____
_____
_____
_____
_____
_____
_____
_____

How was my day? Did I feel good about my performance? What did I learn? Did I have a new insight? What would I do differently?

_____
_____
_____
_____
_____
_____
_____

NOTES AND REFLECTIONS FROM TODAY

What was my energy level today? (lowest to highest) 1 2 3 4 5 6 7 8 9 10

If not a "10", what will I do tomorrow to make it closer to a "10"? _____

I ate my frog today: Yes   No

What Time? _____

I did my new habit: Yes   No

What Time? _____

FOR TOMORROW

_____
_____
_____
_____

"Believe in yourself! Have faith in your abilities! Without a humble but reasonable confidence in your own powers you cannot be successful or happy."
— Norman Vincent Peale

WEEKLY CHECK-INS
WEEK 6

The Purpose of the Weekly Check-In is to...

1) Check-in with your progress throughout the week.

2) Re-focus for the upcoming week.

3) Get inspired for the future.

THE CHECK-IN

What have I accomplished since last week? What were the two most important things that I learned this week? Is there anything that I would have done differently? If so, what?

_____
_____
_____
_____
_____

What are my wins or victories since last week?

_____
_____
_____

What's the highlight (or low-light) of my week?

_____
_____
_____

What am I thankful for this week?

_____
_____
_____

The place I feel stuck is

_____
_____
_____

In which area(s) did I grow the most last week?

Mental Health

Spiritual Health

Career Health

Physical Health

Social Health

Family Health

Financial Health

What was my average energy level for the week?

1 2 3 4 5 6 7 8 9 10

What number do I want it to be next week?

1 2 3 4 5 6 7 8 9 10

How often did you eat your frog?

1 2 3 4 5 6 7

On a 1 - 10 scale, 1 being low and 10 being high, how grateful have I been feeling this last week?

1 2 3 4 5 6 7 8 9 10

How did I do with my new habit building/eliminating?

_____
_____
_____

RE-FOCUS WEEK 6

Every week, we will be re-focusing on our future life. So, take a moment and fill this in again. There will be a few questions after you finish.

If there were no rules, and I could not fail, what would my life be like?

Describe your future life in detail and in writing...

_____
_____
_____
_____
_____
_____
_____
_____

When you wrote this out again, how did you feel? Were you excited? Were you bored? Did your vision evolve? Was it different than before? Was there more detail or less? Did you even do this exercise? If not, how come?

_____
_____
_____

Look through your future life. Now, fill in the blank...

If I only accomplish _____ next week, my future life would surely come to be.

This is your Primary Objective for the next week.

Take a moment and fill in the days of the week for the next week.

Go on to Day 43 and be amazing!

Life Alchemy 1.0

DAILY PREVIEW
DAY 43

M T W T F S S

Date: _____

MY PRIMARY OBJECTIVE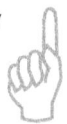

The most important thing I can do today to take me a step closer to my Primary Objective is _____ .

The most important thing I can do today to take me a step closer to my Primary Objective is _____ .

The most important thing I can do today to take me a step closer to my Primary Objective is _____ .

The most important thing I can do today to take me a step closer to my Primary Objective is _____ .

My new habit I'm developing (eliminating) is... _____

MORNING THOUGHTS AND INSPIRATIONS

My biggest frog to eat today...
_____

ACTION STEPS FOR TODAY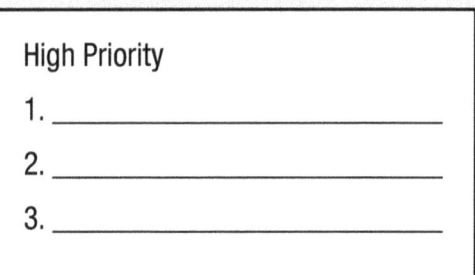

High Priority
1. _____
2. _____
3. _____

Medium Priority
1. _____
2. _____
3. _____

Low Priority
_____
_____
_____
_____
_____
_____

In which area(s) do I want to improve the most today?

Mental Health

Spiritual Health

Career Health

Physical Health

Social Health

Family Health

Financial Health

Weekly Goal Focus:

DAILY REVIEW
DAY 43

Today I am grateful for...

_____
_____
_____
_____
_____
_____
_____
_____

How was my day? Did I feel good about my performance? What did I learn? Did I have a new insight? What would I do differently?

_____
_____
_____
_____
_____
_____
_____
_____

NOTES AND REFLECTIONS FROM TODAY

What was my energy level today? (lowest to highest)   1 2 3 4 5 6 7 8 9 10

If not a "10", what will I do tomorrow to make it closer to a "10"? _____

I ate my frog today: Yes   No

What Time? _____

I did my new habit: Yes   No

What Time? _____

FOR TOMORROW

_____
_____
_____
_____

"Successful and unsuccessful people do not vary greatly in their abilities. They vary in their desires to reach their potential."

John Maxwell

DAILY PREVIEW
DAY 44

M T W T F S S

Date: _____

MY PRIMARY OBJECTIVE

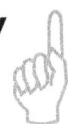

The most important thing I can do today to take me a step closer to my Primary Objective is _____.

The most important thing I can do today to take me a step closer to my Primary Objective is _____.

The most important thing I can do today to take me a step closer to my Primary Objective is _____.

The most important thing I can do today to take me a step closer to my Primary Objective is _____.

My new habit I'm developing (eliminating) is... _____

MORNING THOUGHTS AND INSPIRATIONS

My biggest frog to eat today...
_____

ACTION STEPS FOR TODAY

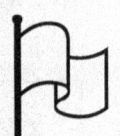

High Priority
1. _____
2. _____
3. _____

Medium Priority
1. _____
2. _____
3. _____

Low Priority
_____
_____
_____
_____
_____
_____

In which area(s) do I want to improve the most today?

Mental Health

Spiritual Health

Career Health

Physical Health

Social Health

Family Health

Financial Health

Weekly Goal Focus:

DAILY REVIEW
DAY 44

Today I am grateful for...

_____
_____
_____
_____
_____
_____
_____

How was my day? Did I feel good about my performance? What did I learn? Did I have a new insight? What would I do differently?

_____
_____
_____
_____
_____
_____
_____

NOTES AND REFLECTIONS FROM TODAY

What was my energy level today? (lowest to highest) 1 2 3 4 5 6 7 8 9 10

If not a "10", what will I do tomorrow to make it closer to a "10"? _____

I ate my frog today: Yes No

What Time? _____

I did my new habit: Yes No

What Time? _____

FOR TOMORROW

_____
_____
_____
_____

"Thinking should become your capital asset, no matter whatever ups and downs you come across in your life."

— Dr. APJ Kalam

Life Alchemy 1.0

DAILY PREVIEW
DAY 45

M T W T F S S

Date: _____

MY PRIMARY OBJECTIVE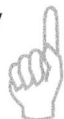

The most important thing I can do today to take me a step closer to my Primary Objective is _____.

The most important thing I can do today to take me a step closer to my Primary Objective is _____.

The most important thing I can do today to take me a step closer to my Primary Objective is _____.

The most important thing I can do today to take me a step closer to my Primary Objective is _____.

My new habit I'm developing (eliminating) is... _____

MORNING THOUGHTS AND INSPIRATIONS

My biggest frog to eat today...
_____

ACTION STEPS FOR TODAY

High Priority
1. _____
2. _____
3. _____

Medium Priority
1. _____
2. _____
3. _____

Low Priority
_____
_____
_____
_____
_____
_____

In which area(s) do I want to improve the most today?

Mental Health

Spiritual Health

Career Health

Physical Health

Social Health

Family Health

Financial Health

Weekly Goal Focus:

DAILY REVIEW
DAY 45

Today I am grateful for...

_____
_____
_____
_____
_____
_____
_____
_____

How was my day? Did I feel good about my performance? What did I learn? Did I have a new insight? What would I do differently?

_____
_____
_____
_____
_____
_____
_____

NOTES AND REFLECTIONS FROM TODAY

What was my energy level today? (lowest to highest) 1 2 3 4 5 6 7 8 9 10

If not a "10", what will I do tomorrow to make it closer to a "10"? _____

I ate my frog today: Yes   No

What Time? _____

I did my new habit: Yes   No

What Time? _____

FOR TOMORROW

_____
_____
_____
_____

"All progress takes place outside the comfort zone."

Michael John Bobak

Life Alchemy 1.0

DAILY PREVIEW
DAY 46

M T W T F S S

Date: _____

MY PRIMARY OBJECTIVE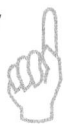

[   ]

The most important thing I can do today to take me a step closer to my Primary Objective is _____.

The most important thing I can do today to take me a step closer to my Primary Objective is _____.

The most important thing I can do today to take me a step closer to my Primary Objective is _____.

The most important thing I can do today to take me a step closer to my Primary Objective is _____.

My new habit I'm developing (eliminating) is... _____

MORNING THOUGHTS AND INSPIRATIONS

My biggest frog to eat today...
_____

ACTION STEPS FOR TODAY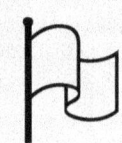

High Priority
1. _____
2. _____
3. _____

Medium Priority
1. _____
2. _____
3. _____

Low Priority
_____
_____
_____
_____
_____
_____

In which area(s) do I want to improve the most today?

Mental Health

Spiritual Health

Career Health

Physical Health

Social Health

Family Health

Financial Health

Weekly Goal Focus:

DAILY REVIEW
DAY 46

Today I am grateful for...

_____
_____
_____
_____
_____
_____
_____
_____

How was my day? Did I feel good about my performance? What did I learn? Did I have a new insight? What would I do differently?

_____
_____
_____
_____
_____
_____
_____
_____

NOTES AND REFLECTIONS FROM TODAY

What was my energy level today? (lowest to highest) 1 2 3 4 5 6 7 8 9 10

If not a "10", what will I do tomorrow to make it closer to a "10"? _____

I ate my frog today: Yes   No

What Time? _____

I did my new habit: Yes   No

What Time? _____

FOR TOMORROW

_____
_____
_____
_____

"People often say that motivation doesn't last. Well, neither does bathing – that's why we recommend it daily."

Zig Ziglar

Life Alchemy 1.0

DAILY PREVIEW
DAY 47

M T W T F S S

Date: _____

MY PRIMARY OBJECTIVE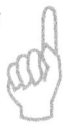

The most important thing I can do today to take me a step closer to my Primary Objective is _____.

The most important thing I can do today to take me a step closer to my Primary Objective is _____.

The most important thing I can do today to take me a step closer to my Primary Objective is _____.

The most important thing I can do today to take me a step closer to my Primary Objective is _____.

My new habit I'm developing (eliminating) is... _____

MORNING THOUGHTS AND INSPIRATIONS

My biggest frog to eat today...
_____

ACTION STEPS FOR TODAY

High Priority
1. _____
2. _____
3. _____

Medium Priority
1. _____
2. _____
3. _____

Low Priority
_____
_____
_____
_____
_____
_____

In which area(s) do I want to improve the most today?

Mental Health

Spiritual Health

Career Health

Physical Health

Social Health

Family Health

Financial Health

Weekly Goal Focus:

DAILY REVIEW
DAY 47

Today I am grateful for...

_____
_____
_____
_____
_____
_____
_____
_____

How was my day? Did I feel good about my performance? What did I learn? Did I have a new insight? What would I do differently?

_____
_____
_____
_____
_____
_____
_____
_____

NOTES AND REFLECTIONS FROM TODAY

What was my energy level today? (lowest to highest) 1 2 3 4 5 6 7 8 9 10

If not a "10", what will I do tomorrow to make it closer to a "10"? _____

I ate my frog today: Yes   No

What Time? _____

I did my new habit: Yes   No

What Time? _____

FOR TOMORROW

_____
_____
_____
_____

"The first step toward success is taken when you refuse to be a captive of the environment in which you first find yourself."

Mark Caine

Life Alchemy 1.0

DAILY PREVIEW
DAY 48

M T W T F S S

Date: _____

MY PRIMARY OBJECTIVE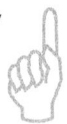

The most important thing I can do today to take me a step closer to my Primary Objective is _____.

The most important thing I can do today to take me a step closer to my Primary Objective is _____.

The most important thing I can do today to take me a step closer to my Primary Objective is _____.

The most important thing I can do today to take me a step closer to my Primary Objective is _____.

My new habit I'm developing (eliminating) is... _____

MORNING THOUGHTS AND INSPIRATIONS

My biggest frog to eat today...
_____

ACTION STEPS FOR TODAY

High Priority
1. _____
2. _____
3. _____

Medium Priority
1. _____
2. _____
3. _____

Low Priority
_____
_____
_____
_____
_____
_____

In which area(s) do I want to improve the most today?

Mental Health

Spiritual Health

Career Health

Physical Health

Social Health

Family Health

Financial Health

Weekly Goal Focus:

DAILY REVIEW
DAY 48

Today I am grateful for...

How was my day? Did I feel good about my performance? What did I learn? Did I have a new insight? What would I do differently?

NOTES AND REFLECTIONS FROM TODAY

What was my energy level today? (lowest to highest) 1 2 3 4 5 6 7 8 9 10

If not a "10", what will I do tomorrow to make it closer to a "10"? _____

I ate my frog today: Yes   No

I did my new habit: Yes   No

What Time? _____

What Time? _____

FOR TOMORROW

"Whenever you find yourself on the side of the majority, it is time to pause and reflect."

Mark Twain

Life Alchemy 1.0

DAILY PREVIEW
DAY 49

M T W T F S S

Date: _____

MY PRIMARY OBJECTIVE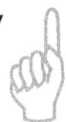

The most important thing I can do today to take me a step closer to my Primary Objective is _____ .

The most important thing I can do today to take me a step closer to my Primary Objective is _____ .

The most important thing I can do today to take me a step closer to my Primary Objective is _____ .

The most important thing I can do today to take me a step closer to my Primary Objective is _____ .

My new habit I'm developing (eliminating) is... _____

MORNING THOUGHTS AND INSPIRATIONS

My biggest frog to eat today...
_____

ACTION STEPS FOR TODAY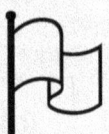

High Priority
1. _____
2. _____
3. _____

Medium Priority
1. _____
2. _____
3. _____

Low Priority
_____
_____
_____
_____
_____
_____

In which area(s) do I want to improve the most today?

Mental Health

Spiritual Health

Career Health

Physical Health

Social Health

Family Health

Financial Health

114

Weekly Goal Focus:

DAILY REVIEW
DAY 49

Today I am grateful for...

_____
_____
_____
_____
_____
_____
_____
_____

How was my day? Did I feel good about my performance? What did I learn? Did I have a new insight? What would I do differently?

_____
_____
_____
_____
_____
_____
_____
_____

NOTES AND REFLECTIONS FROM TODAY

What was my energy level today? (lowest to highest) 1 2 3 4 5 6 7 8 9 10

If not a "10", what will I do tomorrow to make it closer to a "10"? _____

I ate my frog today: Yes   No

What Time? _____

I did my new habit: Yes   No

What Time? _____

FOR TOMORROW

_____
_____
_____
_____

"If you don't design your own life plan, chances are you'll fall into someone else's plan. And guess what they have planned for you? Not much."

Jim Rohn

Life Alchemy 1.0

WEEKLY CHECK-INS
WEEK 7

The Purpose of the Weekly Check-In is to...

1) *Check-in with your progress throughout the week.*

2) *Re-focus for the upcoming week.*

3) *Get inspired for the future.*

THE CHECK-IN

What have I accomplished since last week? What were the two most important things that I learned this week? Is there anything that I would have done differently? If so, what?

_____
_____
_____
_____

What are my wins or victories since last week?

_____
_____
_____

What's the highlight (or low-light) of my week?

_____
_____
_____

What am I thankful for this week?

_____
_____
_____

The place I feel stuck is

_____
_____
_____

In which area(s) did I grow the most last week?

Mental Health

Spiritual Health

Career Health

Physical Health

Social Health

Family Health

Financial Health

What was my average energy level for the week?

1 2 3 4 5 6 7 8 9 10

What number do I want it to be next week?

1 2 3 4 5 6 7 8 9 10

How often did you eat your frog?

1 2 3 4 5 6 7

On a 1 - 10 scale, 1 being low and 10 being high, how grateful have I been feeling this last week?

1 2 3 4 5 6 7 8 9 10

How did I do with my new habit building/eliminating?

_____
_____
_____

RE-FOCUS WEEK 7

Every week, we will be re-focusing on our future life. So, take a moment and fill this in again. There will be a few questions after you finish.

If there were no rules, and I could not fail, what would my life be like?

Describe your future life in detail and in writing...

_____
_____
_____
_____
_____
_____
_____

When you wrote this out again, how did you feel? Were you excited? Were you bored? Did your vision evolve? Was it different than before? Was there more detail or less? Did you even do this exercise? If not, how come?

_____
_____
_____

Look through your future life. Now, fill in the blank...

If I only accomplish _____ next week, my future life would surely come to be.

This is your Primary Objective for the next week.

Take a moment and fill in the days of the week for the next week.

Go on to Day 50 and be amazing!

Life Alchemy 1.0

DAILY PREVIEW
DAY 50

M T W T F S S

Date: _____

MY PRIMARY OBJECTIVE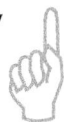

[   ]

The most important thing I can do today to take me a step closer to my Primary Objective is _____ .

The most important thing I can do today to take me a step closer to my Primary Objective is _____ .

The most important thing I can do today to take me a step closer to my Primary Objective is _____ .

The most important thing I can do today to take me a step closer to my Primary Objective is _____ .

My new habit I'm developing (eliminating) is... _____

MORNING THOUGHTS AND INSPIRATIONS

My biggest frog to eat today...
_____

ACTION STEPS FOR TODAY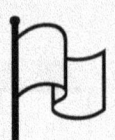

High Priority
1. _____
2. _____
3. _____

Medium Priority
1. _____
2. _____
3. _____

Low Priority
_____
_____
_____
_____
_____
_____

In which area(s) do I want to improve the most today?

Mental Health

Spiritual Health

Career Health

Physical Health

Social Health

Family Health

Financial Health

Weekly Goal Focus:

DAILY REVIEW
DAY 50

Today I am grateful for...

_____
_____
_____
_____
_____
_____
_____

How was my day? Did I feel good about my performance? What did I learn? Did I have a new insight? What would I do differently?

_____
_____
_____
_____
_____
_____
_____

NOTES AND REFLECTIONS FROM TODAY

What was my energy level today? (lowest to highest) 1 2 3 4 5 6 7 8 9 10

If not a "10", what will I do tomorrow to make it closer to a "10"? _____

I ate my frog today: Yes   No

What Time? _____

I did my new habit: Yes   No

What Time? _____

FOR TOMORROW

_____
_____
_____
_____

"If you want to make a permanent change, stop focusing on the size of your problems and start focusing on the size of you!"

T. Harv Eker

Life Alchemy 1.0

DAILY PREVIEW
DAY 51

M T W T F S S

Date: _____

MY PRIMARY OBJECTIVE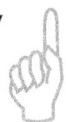

_____

The most important thing I can do today to take me a step closer to my Primary Objective is _____ .

The most important thing I can do today to take me a step closer to my Primary Objective is _____ .

The most important thing I can do today to take me a step closer to my Primary Objective is _____ .

The most important thing I can do today to take me a step closer to my Primary Objective is _____ .

My new habit I'm developing (eliminating) is... _____

MORNING THOUGHTS AND INSPIRATIONS

My biggest frog to eat today...
_____

ACTION STEPS FOR TODAY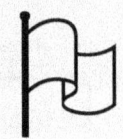

High Priority
1. _____
2. _____
3. _____

Medium Priority
1. _____
2. _____
3. _____

Low Priority
_____
_____
_____
_____
_____
_____

In which area(s) do I want to improve the most today?

Mental Health

Spiritual Health

Career Health

Physical Health

Social Health

Family Health

Financial Health

Weekly Goal Focus:

DAILY REVIEW
DAY 51

Today I am grateful for...

_____
_____
_____
_____
_____
_____
_____
_____

How was my day? Did I feel good about my performance? What did I learn? Did I have a new insight? What would I do differently?

_____
_____
_____
_____
_____
_____
_____
_____

NOTES AND REFLECTIONS FROM TODAY

What was my energy level today? (lowest to highest)   1 2 3 4 5 6 7 8 9 10

If not a "10", what will I do tomorrow to make it closer to a "10"? _____

I ate my frog today: Yes   No

What Time? _____

I did my new habit: Yes   No

What Time? _____

FOR TOMORROW

_____
_____
_____
_____

"In my experience, there is only one motivation, and that is desire. No reasons or principle contain it or stand against it."
— Jane Smiley

DAILY PREVIEW
DAY 52

M T W T F S S

Date: _____

MY PRIMARY OBJECTIVE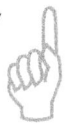

The most important thing I can do today to take me a step closer to my Primary Objective is _____.

The most important thing I can do today to take me a step closer to my Primary Objective is _____.

The most important thing I can do today to take me a step closer to my Primary Objective is _____.

The most important thing I can do today to take me a step closer to my Primary Objective is _____.

My new habit I'm developing (eliminating) is... _____

MORNING THOUGHTS AND INSPIRATIONS

My biggest frog to eat today...
_____

ACTION STEPS FOR TODAY 🏳

High Priority
1. _____
2. _____
3. _____

Medium Priority
1. _____
2. _____
3. _____

Low Priority
_____
_____
_____
_____
_____
_____

In which area(s) do I want to improve the most today?

Mental Health

Spiritual Health

Career Health

Physical Health

Social Health

Family Health

Financial Health

Weekly Goal Focus:

DAILY REVIEW
DAY 52

Today I am grateful for...

_____
_____
_____
_____
_____
_____
_____
_____

How was my day? Did I feel good about my performance? What did I learn? Did I have a new insight? What would I do differently?

_____
_____
_____
_____
_____
_____
_____

NOTES AND REFLECTIONS FROM TODAY

What was my energy level today? (lowest to highest) 1 2 3 4 5 6 7 8 9 10

If not a "10", what will I do tomorrow to make it closer to a "10"? _____

I ate my frog today: Yes   No

What Time? _____

I did my new habit: Yes   No

What Time? _____

FOR TOMORROW

_____
_____
_____
_____

"You must expect great things of yourself before you can do them."

Michael Jordan

Life Alchemy 1.0

DAILY PREVIEW
DAY 53

M T W T F S S

Date: _____

MY PRIMARY OBJECTIVE

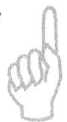

_____

The most important thing I can do today to take me a step closer to my Primary Objective is _____.

The most important thing I can do today to take me a step closer to my Primary Objective is _____.

The most important thing I can do today to take me a step closer to my Primary Objective is _____.

The most important thing I can do today to take me a step closer to my Primary Objective is _____.

My new habit I'm developing (eliminating) is... _____

MORNING THOUGHTS AND INSPIRATIONS

My biggest frog to eat today...
_____

ACTION STEPS FOR TODAY

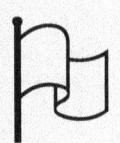

High Priority
1. _____
2. _____
3. _____

Medium Priority
1. _____
2. _____
3. _____

Low Priority
_____
_____
_____
_____
_____
_____

In which area(s) do I want to improve the most today?

Mental Health

Spiritual Health

Career Health

Physical Health

Social Health

Family Health

Financial Health

Weekly Goal Focus:

DAILY REVIEW
DAY 53

Today I am grateful for...

_____
_____
_____
_____
_____
_____
_____
_____

How was my day? Did I feel good about my performance? What did I learn? Did I have a new insight? What would I do differently?

_____
_____
_____
_____
_____
_____
_____

NOTES AND REFLECTIONS FROM TODAY

What was my energy level today? (lowest to highest)   1 2 3 4 5 6 7 8 9 10

If not a "10", what will I do tomorrow to make it closer to a "10"? _____

I ate my frog today: Yes   No

What Time? _____

I did my new habit: Yes   No

What Time? _____

FOR TOMORROW

_____
_____
_____
_____

*"Motivation is what gets you started.
Habit is what keeps you going."*

Jim Ryun

Life Alchemy 1.0

DAILY PREVIEW
DAY 54

M T W T F S S

Date: _____

MY PRIMARY OBJECTIVE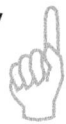

[_____]

The most important thing I can do today to take me a step closer to my Primary Objective is _____.

The most important thing I can do today to take me a step closer to my Primary Objective is _____.

The most important thing I can do today to take me a step closer to my Primary Objective is _____.

The most important thing I can do today to take me a step closer to my Primary Objective is _____.

My new habit I'm developing (eliminating) is... _____

MORNING THOUGHTS AND INSPIRATIONS

My biggest frog to eat today...
_____

ACTION STEPS FOR TODAY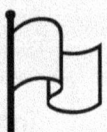

High Priority
1. _____
2. _____
3. _____

Medium Priority
1. _____
2. _____
3. _____

Low Priority
_____
_____
_____
_____
_____
_____

In which area(s) do I want to improve the most today?

Mental Health

Spiritual Health

Career Health

Physical Health

Social Health

Family Health

Financial Health

126

DAILY REVIEW
DAY 54

Weekly Goal Focus:

Today I am grateful for...

_____
_____
_____
_____
_____
_____
_____
_____

How was my day? Did I feel good about my performance? What did I learn? Did I have a new insight? What would I do differently?

_____
_____
_____
_____
_____
_____
_____
_____

NOTES AND REFLECTIONS FROM TODAY

What was my energy level today? (lowest to highest)   1 2 3 4 5 6 7 8 9 10

If not a "10", what will I do tomorrow to make it closer to a "10"? _____

I ate my frog today: Yes   No

What Time? _____

I did my new habit: Yes   No

What Time? _____

FOR TOMORROW

_____
_____
_____
_____

"You've got to get up every morning with determination if you're going to go to bed with satisfaction."

— *George Lorimer*

Life Alchemy 1.0

DAILY PREVIEW
DAY 55

M T W T F S S

Date: _____

MY PRIMARY OBJECTIVE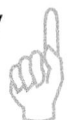

_____

The most important thing I can do today to take me a step closer to my Primary Objective is _____.

The most important thing I can do today to take me a step closer to my Primary Objective is _____.

The most important thing I can do today to take me a step closer to my Primary Objective is _____.

The most important thing I can do today to take me a step closer to my Primary Objective is _____.

My new habit I'm developing (eliminating) is... _____

MORNING THOUGHTS AND INSPIRATIONS

My biggest frog to eat today...
_____

ACTION STEPS FOR TODAY

High Priority
1. _____
2. _____
3. _____

Medium Priority
1. _____
2. _____
3. _____

Low Priority
_____
_____
_____
_____
_____
_____

In which area(s) do I want to improve the most today?

Mental Health

Spiritual Health

Career Health

Physical Health

Social Health

Family Health

Financial Health

Weekly Goal Focus:

DAILY REVIEW
DAY 55

Today I am grateful for...

How was my day? Did I feel good about my performance? What did I learn? Did I have a new insight? What would I do differently?

NOTES AND REFLECTIONS FROM TODAY

What was my energy level today? (lowest to highest)   1 2 3 4 5 6 7 8 9 10

If not a "10", what will I do tomorrow to make it closer to a "10"? _____

I ate my frog today: Yes   No   I did my new habit: Yes   No

What Time? _____   What Time? _____

FOR TOMORROW

"To accomplish great things, we must not only act, but also dream, not only plan, but also believe."

— Anatole France

Life Alchemy 1.0   129

DAILY PREVIEW
DAY 56

M T W T F S S

Date: _____

MY PRIMARY OBJECTIVE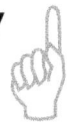

The most important thing I can do today to take me a step closer to my Primary Objective is _____.

The most important thing I can do today to take me a step closer to my Primary Objective is _____.

The most important thing I can do today to take me a step closer to my Primary Objective is _____.

The most important thing I can do today to take me a step closer to my Primary Objective is _____.

My new habit I'm developing (eliminating) is... _____

MORNING THOUGHTS AND INSPIRATIONS

My biggest frog to eat today...
_____

ACTION STEPS FOR TODAY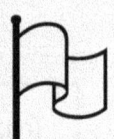

High Priority
1. _____
2. _____
3. _____

Medium Priority
1. _____
2. _____
3. _____

Low Priority
_____
_____
_____
_____
_____
_____

In which area(s) do I want to improve the most today?

Mental Health

Spiritual Health

Career Health

Physical Health

Social Health

Family Health

Financial Health

Weekly Goal Focus:

DAILY REVIEW
DAY 56

Today I am grateful for...

_____
_____
_____
_____
_____
_____
_____
_____

How was my day? Did I feel good about my performance? What did I learn? Did I have a new insight? What would I do differently?

_____
_____
_____
_____
_____
_____
_____
_____

NOTES AND REFLECTIONS FROM TODAY

What was my energy level today? (lowest to highest)   1 2 3 4 5 6 7 8 9 10

If not a "10", what will I do tomorrow to make it closer to a "10"? _____

I ate my frog today: Yes   No   I did my new habit: Yes   No

What Time? _____   What Time? _____

FOR TOMORROW

_____
_____
_____
_____

"It is better to fail in originality than to succeed in imitation."

— Herman Melville

WEEKLY CHECK-INS
WEEK 8

The Purpose of the Weekly Check-In is to...

1) *Check-in with your progress throughout the week.*

2) *Re-focus for the upcoming week.*

3) *Get inspired for the future.*

THE CHECK-IN

What have I accomplished since last week? What were the two most important things that I learned this week? Is there anything that I would have done differently? If so, what?

_____
_____
_____
_____
_____

What are my wins or victories since last week?

_____
_____
_____

What's the highlight (or low-light) of my week?

_____
_____
_____

What am I thankful for this week?

_____
_____
_____

The place I feel stuck is

_____
_____
_____

In which area(s) did I grow the most last week?

Mental Health

Spiritual Health

Career Health

Physical Health

Social Health

Family Health

Financial Health

What was my average energy level for the week?

1 2 3 4 5 6 7 8 9 10

What number do I want it to be next week?

1 2 3 4 5 6 7 8 9 10

How often did you eat your frog?

1 2 3 4 5 6 7

On a 1 - 10 scale, 1 being low and 10 being high, how grateful have I been feeling this last week?

1 2 3 4 5 6 7 8 9 10

How did I do with my new habit building/eliminating?

_____
_____
_____

RE-FOCUS
WEEK 8

Every week, we will be re-focusing on our future life. So, take a moment and fill this in again. There will be a few questions after you finish.

If there were no rules, and I could not fail, what would my life be like?

Describe your future life in detail and in writing...

_____
_____
_____
_____
_____
_____
_____

When you wrote this out again, how did you feel? Were you excited? Were you bored? Did your vision evolve? Was it different than before? Was there more detail or less? Did you even do this exercise? If not, how come?

_____
_____
_____

Look through your future life. Now, fill in the blank...

If I only accomplish _____ next week, my future life would surely come to be.

This is your Primary Objective for the next week.

Take a moment and fill in the days of the week for the next week.

Go on to Day 57 and be amazing!

Life Alchemy 1.0

DAILY PREVIEW
DAY 57

M T W T F S S

Date: _____

MY PRIMARY OBJECTIVE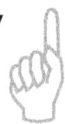

The most important thing I can do today to take me a step closer to my Primary Objective is _____.

The most important thing I can do today to take me a step closer to my Primary Objective is _____.

The most important thing I can do today to take me a step closer to my Primary Objective is _____.

The most important thing I can do today to take me a step closer to my Primary Objective is _____.

My new habit I'm developing (eliminating) is... _____

MORNING THOUGHTS AND INSPIRATIONS

My biggest frog to eat today...
_____

ACTION STEPS FOR TODAY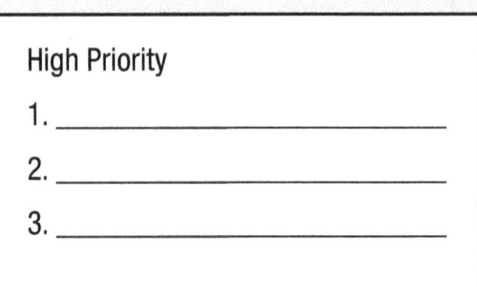

High Priority
1. _____
2. _____
3. _____

Medium Priority
1. _____
2. _____
3. _____

Low Priority
_____
_____
_____
_____
_____
_____

In which area(s) do I want to improve the most today?

Mental Health

Spiritual Health

Career Health

Physical Health

Social Health

Family Health

Financial Health

Weekly Goal Focus:

DAILY REVIEW
DAY 57

Today I am grateful for...

How was my day? Did I feel good about my performance? What did I learn? Did I have a new insight? What would I do differently?

NOTES AND REFLECTIONS FROM TODAY

What was my energy level today? (lowest to highest) 1 2 3 4 5 6 7 8 9 10

If not a "10", what will I do tomorrow to make it closer to a "10"? _____

I ate my frog today: Yes   No

I did my new habit: Yes   No

What Time? _____

What Time? _____

FOR TOMORROW

"Don't let what you cannot do interfere with what you can do."

John R. Wooden

Life Alchemy 1.0

DAILY PREVIEW
DAY 58

M T W T F S S

Date: _____

MY PRIMARY OBJECTIVE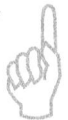

The most important thing I can do today to take me a step closer to my Primary Objective is _____.

The most important thing I can do today to take me a step closer to my Primary Objective is _____.

The most important thing I can do today to take me a step closer to my Primary Objective is _____.

The most important thing I can do today to take me a step closer to my Primary Objective is _____.

My new habit I'm developing (eliminating) is... _____

MORNING THOUGHTS AND INSPIRATIONS

My biggest frog to eat today...
_____

ACTION STEPS FOR TODAY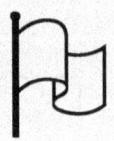

High Priority
1. _____
2. _____
3. _____

Medium Priority
1. _____
2. _____
3. _____

Low Priority
_____
_____
_____
_____
_____
_____

In which area(s) do I want to improve the most today?

Mental Health

Spiritual Health

Career Health

Physical Health

Social Health

Family Health

Financial Health

Weekly Goal Focus:

DAILY REVIEW
DAY 58

Today I am grateful for...

How was my day? Did I feel good about my performance? What did I learn? Did I have a new insight? What would I do differently?

NOTES AND REFLECTIONS FROM TODAY

What was my energy level today? (lowest to highest) 1 2 3 4 5 6 7 8 9 10

If not a "10", what will I do tomorrow to make it closer to a "10"? _____

I ate my frog today: Yes   No

What Time? _____

I did my new habit: Yes   No

What Time? _____

FOR TOMORROW

"If you don't build your dream, someone else will hire you to help them build theirs."

Dhirubhai Ambani

Life Alchemy 1.0

DAILY PREVIEW
DAY 59

M T W T F S S

Date: _____

MY PRIMARY OBJECTIVE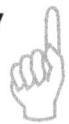

The most important thing I can do today to take me a step closer to my Primary Objective is _____ .

The most important thing I can do today to take me a step closer to my Primary Objective is _____ .

The most important thing I can do today to take me a step closer to my Primary Objective is _____ .

The most important thing I can do today to take me a step closer to my Primary Objective is _____ .

My new habit I'm developing (eliminating) is… _____

MORNING THOUGHTS AND INSPIRATIONS

My biggest frog to eat today…
_____

ACTION STEPS FOR TODAY

High Priority
1. _____
2. _____
3. _____

Medium Priority
1. _____
2. _____
3. _____

Low Priority
_____
_____
_____
_____
_____
_____

In which area(s) do I want to improve the most today?

Mental Health

Spiritual Health

Career Health

Physical Health

Social Health

Family Health

Financial Health

Weekly Goal Focus:

DAILY REVIEW
DAY 59

Today I am grateful for...

_____
_____
_____
_____
_____
_____
_____
_____

How was my day? Did I feel good about my performance? What did I learn? Did I have a new insight? What would I do differently?

_____
_____
_____
_____
_____
_____
_____

NOTES AND REFLECTIONS FROM TODAY

What was my energy level today? (lowest to highest) 1 2 3 4 5 6 7 8 9 10

If not a "10", what will I do tomorrow to make it closer to a "10"? _____

I ate my frog today: Yes   No   I did my new habit: Yes   No

What Time? _____   What Time? _____

FOR TOMORROW

_____
_____
_____
_____

"You may have to fight a battle more than once to win it."

Margaret Thatcher

DAILY PREVIEW
DAY 60

M T W T F S S

Date: _____

MY PRIMARY OBJECTIVE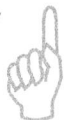

The most important thing I can do today to take me a step closer to my Primary Objective is _____.

The most important thing I can do today to take me a step closer to my Primary Objective is _____.

The most important thing I can do today to take me a step closer to my Primary Objective is _____.

The most important thing I can do today to take me a step closer to my Primary Objective is _____.

My new habit I'm developing (eliminating) is... _____

MORNING THOUGHTS AND INSPIRATIONS

My biggest frog to eat today...
_____

ACTION STEPS FOR TODAY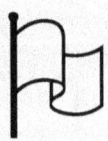

High Priority
1. _____
2. _____
3. _____

Medium Priority
1. _____
2. _____
3. _____

Low Priority
_____
_____
_____
_____
_____
_____

In which area(s) do I want to improve the most today?

Mental Health

Spiritual Health

Career Health

Physical Health

Social Health

Family Health

Financial Health

Weekly Goal Focus:

DAILY REVIEW
DAY 60

Today I am grateful for...

_____
_____
_____
_____
_____
_____
_____
_____

How was my day? Did I feel good about my performance? What did I learn? Did I have a new insight? What would I do differently?

_____
_____
_____
_____
_____
_____
_____

NOTES AND REFLECTIONS FROM TODAY

What was my energy level today? (lowest to highest) 1 2 3 4 5 6 7 8 9 10

If not a "10", what will I do tomorrow to make it closer to a "10"? _____

I ate my frog today: Yes   No

What Time? _____

I did my new habit: Yes   No

What Time? _____

"If you set your goals ridiculously high and it's a failure, you will fail above everyone else's success."

James Cameron

FOR TOMORROW

_____
_____
_____
_____

Life Alchemy 1.0

DAILY PREVIEW
DAY 61

M T W T F S S

Date: _____

MY PRIMARY OBJECTIVE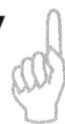

The most important thing I can do today to take me a step closer to my Primary Objective is _____.

The most important thing I can do today to take me a step closer to my Primary Objective is _____.

The most important thing I can do today to take me a step closer to my Primary Objective is _____.

The most important thing I can do today to take me a step closer to my Primary Objective is _____.

My new habit I'm developing (eliminating) is... _____

MORNING THOUGHTS AND INSPIRATIONS

My biggest frog to eat today...
_____

ACTION STEPS FOR TODAY

High Priority
1. _____
2. _____
3. _____

Medium Priority
1. _____
2. _____
3. _____

Low Priority
_____
_____
_____
_____
_____
_____

In which area(s) do I want to improve the most today?

Mental Health

Spiritual Health

Career Health

Physical Health

Social Health

Family Health

Financial Health

Weekly Goal Focus:

DAILY REVIEW
DAY 61

Today I am grateful for...

How was my day? Did I feel good about my performance? What did I learn? Did I have a new insight? What would I do differently?

NOTES AND REFLECTIONS FROM TODAY

What was my energy level today? (lowest to highest) 1 2 3 4 5 6 7 8 9 10

If not a "10", what will I do tomorrow to make it closer to a "10"? _____

I ate my frog today: Yes   No

I did my new habit: Yes   No

What Time? _____

What Time? _____

FOR TOMORROW

"Let him who would enjoy a good future waste none of his present."

— Roger Babson

Life Alchemy 1.0

DAILY PREVIEW
DAY 62

M T W T F S S

Date: _____

MY PRIMARY OBJECTIVE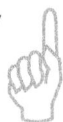

The most important thing I can do today to take me a step closer to my Primary Objective is _____.

The most important thing I can do today to take me a step closer to my Primary Objective is _____.

The most important thing I can do today to take me a step closer to my Primary Objective is _____.

The most important thing I can do today to take me a step closer to my Primary Objective is _____.

My new habit I'm developing (eliminating) is... _____

MORNING THOUGHTS AND INSPIRATIONS

My biggest frog to eat today...
_____

ACTION STEPS FOR TODAY

High Priority
1. _____
2. _____
3. _____

Medium Priority
1. _____
2. _____
3. _____

Low Priority
_____
_____
_____
_____
_____
_____

In which area(s) do I want to improve the most today?

Mental Health

Spiritual Health

Career Health

Physical Health

Social Health

Family Health

Financial Health

Weekly Goal Focus:

DAILY REVIEW
DAY 62

Today I am grateful for...

How was my day? Did I feel good about my performance? What did I learn? Did I have a new insight? What would I do differently?

NOTES AND REFLECTIONS FROM TODAY

What was my energy level today? (lowest to highest)   1 2 3 4 5 6 7 8 9 10

If not a "10", what will I do tomorrow to make it closer to a "10"? _____

I ate my frog today: Yes   No   I did my new habit: Yes   No

What Time? _____   What Time? _____

FOR TOMORROW

"Success is about creating benefit for all and enjoying the process. If you focus on this and adopt this definition, success is yours."

Kelly Kim

Life Alchemy 1.0

DAILY PREVIEW
DAY 63

M T W T F S S

Date: _____

MY PRIMARY OBJECTIVE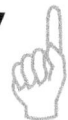

The most important thing I can do today to take me a step closer to my Primary Objective is _____.

The most important thing I can do today to take me a step closer to my Primary Objective is _____.

The most important thing I can do today to take me a step closer to my Primary Objective is _____.

The most important thing I can do today to take me a step closer to my Primary Objective is _____.

My new habit I'm developing (eliminating) is... _____

MORNING THOUGHTS AND INSPIRATIONS

My biggest frog to eat today...
_____

ACTION STEPS FOR TODAY

High Priority
1. _____
2. _____
3. _____

Medium Priority
1. _____
2. _____
3. _____

Low Priority
_____
_____
_____
_____
_____
_____

In which area(s) do I want to improve the most today?

Mental Health

Spiritual Health

Career Health

Physical Health

Social Health

Family Health

Financial Health

Weekly Goal Focus:

DAILY REVIEW
DAY 63

Today I am grateful for...

_____
_____
_____
_____
_____
_____
_____

How was my day? Did I feel good about my performance? What did I learn? Did I have a new insight? What would I do differently?

_____
_____
_____
_____
_____
_____

NOTES AND REFLECTIONS FROM TODAY

What was my energy level today? (lowest to highest)   1 2 3 4 5 6 7 8 9 10

If not a "10", what will I do tomorrow to make it closer to a "10"? _____

I ate my frog today: Yes   No

I did my new habit: Yes   No

What Time? _____

What Time? _____

FOR TOMORROW

_____
_____
_____
_____

"Really it comes down to your philosophy. Do you want to play it safe and be good or do you want to take a chance and be great?"

Jimmy J

Life Alchemy 1.0

WEEKLY CHECK-INS
WEEK 9

The Purpose of the Weekly Check-In is to...

1) Check-in with your progress throughout the week.

2) Re-focus for the upcoming week.

3) Get inspired for the future.

THE CHECK-IN

What have I accomplished since last week? What were the two most important things that I learned this week? Is there anything that I would have done differently? If so, what?

_____
_____
_____
_____
_____

What are my wins or victories since last week?

_____
_____
_____

What's the highlight (or low-light) of my week?

_____
_____
_____

What am I thankful for this week?

_____
_____
_____

The place I feel stuck is

_____
_____
_____

In which area(s) did I grow the most last week?

Mental Health

Spiritual Health

Career Health

Physical Health

Social Health

Family Health

Financial Health

What was my average energy level for the week?

1 2 3 4 5 6 7 8 9 10

What number do I want it to be next week?

1 2 3 4 5 6 7 8 9 10

How often did you eat your frog?

1 2 3 4 5 6 7

On a 1 - 10 scale, 1 being low and 10 being high, how grateful have I been feeling this last week?

1 2 3 4 5 6 7 8 9 10

How did I do with my new habit building/eliminating?

_____
_____
_____

RE-FOCUS WEEK 9

Every week, we will be re-focusing on our future life. So, take a moment and fill this in again. There will be a few questions after you finish.

If there were no rules, and I could not fail, what would my life be like?

Describe your future life in detail and in writing...

_____
_____
_____
_____
_____
_____
_____

When you wrote this out again, how did you feel? Were you excited? Were you bored? Did your vision evolve? Was it different than before? Was there more detail or less? Did you even do this exercise? If not, how come?

_____
_____
_____

Look through your future life. Now, fill in the blank...

If I only accomplish _____ next week, my future life would surely come to be.

This is your Primary Objective for the next week.

Take a moment and fill in the days of the week for the next week.

Go on to Day 64 and be amazing!

Life Alchemy 1.0

DAILY PREVIEW
DAY 64

M T W T F S S

Date: _____

MY PRIMARY OBJECTIVE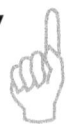

The most important thing I can do today to take me a step closer to my Primary Objective is _____.

The most important thing I can do today to take me a step closer to my Primary Objective is _____.

The most important thing I can do today to take me a step closer to my Primary Objective is _____.

The most important thing I can do today to take me a step closer to my Primary Objective is _____.

My new habit I'm developing (eliminating) is... _____

MORNING THOUGHTS AND INSPIRATIONS

My biggest frog to eat today...
_____

ACTION STEPS FOR TODAY

High Priority
1. _____
2. _____
3. _____

Medium Priority
1. _____
2. _____
3. _____

Low Priority
_____
_____
_____
_____
_____
_____

In which area(s) do I want to improve the most today?

Mental Health

Spiritual Health

Career Health

Physical Health

Social Health

Family Health

Financial Health

Weekly Goal Focus:

DAILY REVIEW
DAY 64

Today I am grateful for...

How was my day? Did I feel good about my performance? What did I learn? Did I have a new insight? What would I do differently?

NOTES AND REFLECTIONS FROM TODAY

What was my energy level today? (lowest to highest)   1 2 3 4 5 6 7 8 9 10

If not a "10", what will I do tomorrow to make it closer to a "10"? _____

I ate my frog today: Yes   No   I did my new habit: Yes   No

What Time? _____   What Time? _____

FOR TOMORROW

"It is our choices that show what we truly are, far more than our abilities."

J. K. Rowling

Life Alchemy 1.0

DAILY PREVIEW
DAY 65

M T W T F S S

Date: _____

MY PRIMARY OBJECTIVE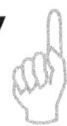

The most important thing I can do today to take me a step closer to my Primary Objective is _____ .

The most important thing I can do today to take me a step closer to my Primary Objective is _____ .

The most important thing I can do today to take me a step closer to my Primary Objective is _____ .

The most important thing I can do today to take me a step closer to my Primary Objective is _____ .

My new habit I'm developing (eliminating) is… _____

MORNING THOUGHTS AND INSPIRATIONS

My biggest frog to eat today...
_____

ACTION STEPS FOR TODAY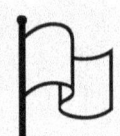

High Priority
1. _____
2. _____
3. _____

Medium Priority
1. _____
2. _____
3. _____

Low Priority
_____
_____
_____
_____
_____
_____

In which area(s) do I want to improve the most today?

Mental Health

Spiritual Health

Career Health

Physical Health

Social Health

Family Health

Financial Health

Weekly Goal Focus:

DAILY REVIEW
DAY 65

Today I am grateful for...

How was my day? Did I feel good about my performance? What did I learn? Did I have a new insight? What would I do differently?

NOTES AND REFLECTIONS FROM TODAY

What was my energy level today? (lowest to highest) 1 2 3 4 5 6 7 8 9 10

If not a "10", what will I do tomorrow to make it closer to a "10"? _____

I ate my frog today: Yes   No

I did my new habit: Yes   No

What Time? _____

What Time? _____

FOR TOMORROW

"If you genuinely want something, don't wait for it – teach yourself to be impatient."

Gurbaksh Chahal

Life Alchemy 1.0

DAILY PREVIEW
DAY 66

M T W T F S S

Date: _____

MY PRIMARY OBJECTIVE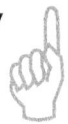

The most important thing I can do today to take me a step closer to my Primary Objective is _____.

The most important thing I can do today to take me a step closer to my Primary Objective is _____.

The most important thing I can do today to take me a step closer to my Primary Objective is _____.

The most important thing I can do today to take me a step closer to my Primary Objective is _____.

My new habit I'm developing (eliminating) is... _____

MORNING THOUGHTS AND INSPIRATIONS

My biggest frog to eat today...
_____

ACTION STEPS FOR TODAY

High Priority
1. _____
2. _____
3. _____

Medium Priority
1. _____
2. _____
3. _____

Low Priority
_____
_____
_____
_____
_____
_____

In which area(s) do I want to improve the most today?

Mental Health

Spiritual Health

Career Health

Physical Health

Social Health

Family Health

Financial Health

Weekly Goal Focus:

DAILY REVIEW
DAY 66

Today I am grateful for...

_____
_____
_____
_____
_____
_____
_____
_____

How was my day? Did I feel good about my performance? What did I learn? Did I have a new insight? What would I do differently?

_____
_____
_____
_____
_____
_____
_____

NOTES AND REFLECTIONS FROM TODAY

What was my energy level today? (lowest to highest) 1 2 3 4 5 6 7 8 9 10

If not a "10", what will I do tomorrow to make it closer to a "10"? _____

I ate my frog today: Yes   No

What Time? _____

I did my new habit: Yes   No

What Time? _____

FOR TOMORROW

_____
_____
_____
_____

"A person is a success if they get up in the morning and gets to bed at night and in between does what he wants to do."

Bob Dylan

Life Alchemy 1.0   155

DAILY PREVIEW
DAY 67

M T W T F S S

Date: _____

MY PRIMARY OBJECTIVE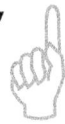

The most important thing I can do today to take me a step closer to my Primary Objective is _____.

The most important thing I can do today to take me a step closer to my Primary Objective is _____.

The most important thing I can do today to take me a step closer to my Primary Objective is _____.

The most important thing I can do today to take me a step closer to my Primary Objective is _____.

My new habit I'm developing (eliminating) is... _____

MORNING THOUGHTS AND INSPIRATIONS

My biggest frog to eat today...
_____

ACTION STEPS FOR TODAY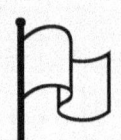

High Priority
1. _____
2. _____
3. _____

Medium Priority
1. _____
2. _____
3. _____

Low Priority
_____
_____
_____
_____
_____
_____

In which area(s) do I want to improve the most today?

Mental Health

Spiritual Health

Career Health

Physical Health

Social Health

Family Health

Financial Health

Weekly Goal Focus:

DAILY REVIEW
DAY 67

Today I am grateful for...

How was my day? Did I feel good about my performance? What did I learn? Did I have a new insight? What would I do differently?

NOTES AND REFLECTIONS FROM TODAY

What was my energy level today? (lowest to highest)   1 2 3 4 5 6 7 8 9 10

If not a "10", what will I do tomorrow to make it closer to a "10"? _____

I ate my frog today: Yes   No   I did my new habit: Yes   No

What Time? _____   What Time? _____

FOR TOMORROW

"Success is not the result of making money; making money is the result of success and success is in direct proportion to our service."

Earl Nightingale

Life Alchemy 1.0

DAILY PREVIEW
DAY 68

M T W T F S S

Date: _____

MY PRIMARY OBJECTIVE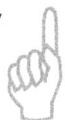

The most important thing I can do today to take me a step closer to my Primary Objective is _____.

The most important thing I can do today to take me a step closer to my Primary Objective is _____.

The most important thing I can do today to take me a step closer to my Primary Objective is _____.

The most important thing I can do today to take me a step closer to my Primary Objective is _____.

My new habit I'm developing (eliminating) is... _____

MORNING THOUGHTS AND INSPIRATIONS

My biggest frog to eat today...
_____

ACTION STEPS FOR TODAY

High Priority
1. _____
2. _____
3. _____

Medium Priority
1. _____
2. _____
3. _____

Low Priority
_____
_____
_____
_____
_____
_____

In which area(s) do I want to improve the most today?

Mental Health

Spiritual Health

Career Health

Physical Health

Social Health

Family Health

Financial Health

Weekly Goal Focus:

DAILY REVIEW
DAY 68

Today I am grateful for...

_____
_____
_____
_____
_____
_____
_____

How was my day? Did I feel good about my performance? What did I learn? Did I have a new insight? What would I do differently?

_____
_____
_____
_____
_____
_____
_____

NOTES AND REFLECTIONS FROM TODAY

What was my energy level today? (lowest to highest)   1 2 3 4 5 6 7 8 9 10

If not a "10", what will I do tomorrow to make it closer to a "10"? _____

I ate my frog today: Yes   No

What Time? _____

I did my new habit: Yes   No

What Time? _____

"Success is a commitment to personal growth on a daily basis."

Tony Robbins

FOR TOMORROW

_____
_____
_____
_____

Life Alchemy 1.0

DAILY PREVIEW
DAY 69

M T W T F S S

Date: _____

MY PRIMARY OBJECTIVE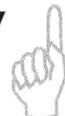

The most important thing I can do today to take me a step closer to my Primary Objective is _____.

The most important thing I can do today to take me a step closer to my Primary Objective is _____.

The most important thing I can do today to take me a step closer to my Primary Objective is _____.

The most important thing I can do today to take me a step closer to my Primary Objective is _____.

My new habit I'm developing (eliminating) is... _____

MORNING THOUGHTS AND INSPIRATIONS

My biggest frog to eat today...
_____

ACTION STEPS FOR TODAY

High Priority
1. _____
2. _____
3. _____

Medium Priority
1. _____
2. _____
3. _____

Low Priority
_____
_____
_____
_____
_____
_____

In which area(s) do I want to improve the most today?

Mental Health

Spiritual Health

Career Health

Physical Health

Social Health

Family Health

Financial Health

Weekly Goal Focus:

DAILY REVIEW
DAY 69

Today I am grateful for...

_____
_____
_____
_____
_____
_____
_____
_____

How was my day? Did I feel good about my performance? What did I learn? Did I have a new insight? What would I do differently?

_____
_____
_____
_____
_____
_____
_____
_____

NOTES AND REFLECTIONS FROM TODAY

What was my energy level today? (lowest to highest)   1 2 3 4 5 6 7 8 9 10

If not a "10", what will I do tomorrow to make it closer to a "10"? _____

I ate my frog today: Yes   No

What Time? _____

I did my new habit: Yes   No

What Time? _____

FOR TOMORROW

_____
_____
_____
_____

"Help others achieve their dreams and you will achieve yours."

Les Brown

Life Alchemy 1.0

DAILY PREVIEW
DAY 70

M T W T F S S

Date: _____

MY PRIMARY OBJECTIVE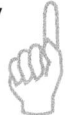

_____

The most important thing I can do today to take me a step closer to my Primary Objective is _____.

The most important thing I can do today to take me a step closer to my Primary Objective is _____.

The most important thing I can do today to take me a step closer to my Primary Objective is _____.

The most important thing I can do today to take me a step closer to my Primary Objective is _____.

My new habit I'm developing (eliminating) is... _____

MORNING THOUGHTS AND INSPIRATIONS

My biggest frog to eat today...
_____

ACTION STEPS FOR TODAY

High Priority
1. _____
2. _____
3. _____

Medium Priority
1. _____
2. _____
3. _____

Low Priority
_____
_____
_____
_____
_____
_____

In which area(s) do I want to improve the most today?

Mental Health

Spiritual Health

Career Health

Physical Health

Social Health

Family Health

Financial Health

Weekly Goal Focus:

DAILY REVIEW
DAY 70

Today I am grateful for...

How was my day? Did I feel good about my performance? What did I learn? Did I have a new insight? What would I do differently?

NOTES AND REFLECTIONS FROM TODAY

What was my energy level today? (lowest to highest) 1 2 3 4 5 6 7 8 9 10

If not a "10", what will I do tomorrow to make it closer to a "10"? _____

I ate my frog today: Yes   No

I did my new habit: Yes   No

What Time? _____

What Time? _____

FOR TOMORROW

"Success is something you attract by the person you become."

Jim Rohn

Life Alchemy 1.0

WEEKLY CHECK-INS
WEEK 10

The Purpose of the Weekly Check-In is to...

1) *Check-in with your progress throughout the week.*

2) *Re-focus for the upcoming week.*

3) *Get inspired for the future.*

THE CHECK-IN

What have I accomplished since last week? What were the two most important things that I learned this week? Is there anything that I would have done differently? If so, what?

___

What are my wins or victories since last week?

___

What's the highlight (or low-light) of my week?

___

What am I thankful for this week?

___

The place I feel stuck is

___

In which area(s) did I grow the most last week?

Mental Health

Spiritual Health

Career Health

Physical Health

Social Health

Family Health

Financial Health

What was my average energy level for the week?

1 2 3 4 5 6 7 8 9 10

What number do I want it to be next week?

1 2 3 4 5 6 7 8 9 10

How often did you eat your frog?

1 2 3 4 5 6 7

On a 1 - 10 scale, 1 being low and 10 being high, how grateful have I been feeling this last week?

1 2 3 4 5 6 7 8 9 10

How did I do with my new habit building/eliminating?

___

RE-FOCUS WEEK 10

Every week, we will be re-focusing on our future life. So, take a moment and fill this in again. There will be a few questions after you finish.

If there were no rules, and I could not fail, what would my life be like?

Describe your future life in detail and in writing...

_____
_____
_____
_____
_____
_____
_____

When you wrote this out again, how did you feel? Were you excited? Were you bored? Did your vision evolve? Was it different than before? Was there more detail or less? Did you even do this exercise? If not, how come?

_____
_____
_____

Look through your future life. Now, fill in the blank...

If I only accomplish _____ next week, my future life would surely come to be.

This is your Primary Objective for the next week.

Take a moment and fill in the days of the week for the next week.

Go on to Day 71 and be amazing!

Life Alchemy 1.0

DAILY PREVIEW
DAY 71

M T W T F S S

Date: _____

MY PRIMARY OBJECTIVE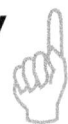

The most important thing I can do today to take me a step closer to my Primary Objective is _____.

The most important thing I can do today to take me a step closer to my Primary Objective is _____.

The most important thing I can do today to take me a step closer to my Primary Objective is _____.

The most important thing I can do today to take me a step closer to my Primary Objective is _____.

My new habit I'm developing (eliminating) is... _____

MORNING THOUGHTS AND INSPIRATIONS

My biggest frog to eat today...
_____

ACTION STEPS FOR TODAY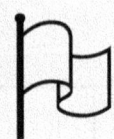

High Priority
1. _____
2. _____
3. _____

Medium Priority
1. _____
2. _____
3. _____

Low Priority
_____
_____
_____
_____
_____
_____

In which area(s) do I want to improve the most today?

Mental Health

Spiritual Health

Career Health

Physical Health

Social Health

Family Health

Financial Health

Weekly Goal Focus:

DAILY REVIEW
DAY 71

Today I am grateful for...

_____
_____
_____
_____
_____
_____
_____
_____

How was my day? Did I feel good about my performance? What did I learn? Did I have a new insight? What would I do differently?

_____
_____
_____
_____
_____
_____
_____
_____

NOTES AND REFLECTIONS FROM TODAY

What was my energy level today? (lowest to highest)   1 2 3 4 5 6 7 8 9 10

If not a "10", what will I do tomorrow to make it closer to a "10"? _____

I ate my frog today: Yes   No

I did my new habit: Yes   No

What Time? _____

What Time? _____

FOR TOMORROW

_____
_____
_____
_____

"Success is a journey, not a destination. The doing is often more important than the outcome."

Arthur Ashe

DAILY PREVIEW
DAY 72

M T W T F S S

Date: _____

MY PRIMARY OBJECTIVE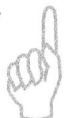

[_____]

The most important thing I can do today to take me a step closer to my Primary Objective is _____.

The most important thing I can do today to take me a step closer to my Primary Objective is _____.

The most important thing I can do today to take me a step closer to my Primary Objective is _____.

The most important thing I can do today to take me a step closer to my Primary Objective is _____.

My new habit I'm developing (eliminating) is... _____

MORNING THOUGHTS AND INSPIRATIONS

My biggest frog to eat today...
_____

ACTION STEPS FOR TODAY

High Priority
1. _____
2. _____
3. _____

Medium Priority
1. _____
2. _____
3. _____

Low Priority
_____
_____
_____
_____
_____
_____

In which area(s) do I want to improve the most today?

Mental Health

Spiritual Health

Career Health

Physical Health

Social Health

Family Health

Financial Health

Weekly Goal Focus:

DAILY REVIEW
DAY 72

Today I am grateful for...

How was my day? Did I feel good about my performance? What did I learn? Did I have a new insight? What would I do differently?

NOTES AND REFLECTIONS FROM TODAY

What was my energy level today? (lowest to highest)   1 2 3 4 5 6 7 8 9 10

If not a "10", what will I do tomorrow to make it closer to a "10"? _____

I ate my frog today: Yes   No

I did my new habit: Yes   No

What Time? _____

What Time? _____

FOR TOMORROW

"Success is achieved by developing our strengths, not by eliminating our weaknesses."

Marilyn vos Savant

Life Alchemy 1.0

DAILY PREVIEW
DAY 73

M T W T F S S

Date: _____

MY PRIMARY OBJECTIVE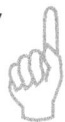

The most important thing I can do today to take me a step closer to my Primary Objective is _____.

The most important thing I can do today to take me a step closer to my Primary Objective is _____.

The most important thing I can do today to take me a step closer to my Primary Objective is _____.

The most important thing I can do today to take me a step closer to my Primary Objective is _____.

My new habit I'm developing (eliminating) is... _____

MORNING THOUGHTS AND INSPIRATIONS

My biggest frog to eat today...
_____

ACTION STEPS FOR TODAY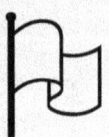

High Priority
1. _____
2. _____
3. _____

Medium Priority
1. _____
2. _____
3. _____

Low Priority
_____
_____
_____
_____
_____
_____

In which area(s) do I want to improve the most today?

Mental Health

Spiritual Health

Career Health

Physical Health

Social Health

Family Health

Financial Health

Weekly Goal Focus:

DAILY REVIEW
DAY 73

Today I am grateful for...

_____
_____
_____
_____
_____
_____
_____
_____

How was my day? Did I feel good about my performance? What did I learn? Did I have a new insight? What would I do differently?

_____
_____
_____
_____
_____
_____
_____
_____

NOTES AND REFLECTIONS FROM TODAY

What was my energy level today? (lowest to highest)   1 2 3 4 5 6 7 8 9 10

If not a "10", what will I do tomorrow to make it closer to a "10"? _____

I ate my frog today: Yes   No

What Time? _____

I did my new habit: Yes   No

What Time? _____

FOR TOMORROW

_____
_____
_____
_____

"The less people speak of their greatness, the more we think of it."

Francis Bacon

Life Alchemy 1.0

DAILY PREVIEW
DAY 74

M T W T F S S

Date: _____

MY PRIMARY OBJECTIVE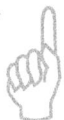

The most important thing I can do today to take me a step closer to my Primary Objective is _____.

The most important thing I can do today to take me a step closer to my Primary Objective is _____.

The most important thing I can do today to take me a step closer to my Primary Objective is _____.

The most important thing I can do today to take me a step closer to my Primary Objective is _____.

My new habit I'm developing (eliminating) is... _____

MORNING THOUGHTS AND INSPIRATIONS

My biggest frog to eat today...
_____

ACTION STEPS FOR TODAY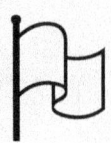

High Priority
1. _____
2. _____
3. _____

Medium Priority
1. _____
2. _____
3. _____

Low Priority
_____
_____
_____
_____
_____
_____

In which area(s) do I want to improve the most today?

Mental Health

Spiritual Health

Career Health

Physical Health

Social Health

Family Health

Financial Health

Weekly Goal Focus:

DAILY REVIEW
DAY 74

Today I am grateful for...

How was my day? Did I feel good about my performance? What did I learn? Did I have a new insight? What would I do differently?

NOTES AND REFLECTIONS FROM TODAY

What was my energy level today? (lowest to highest) 1 2 3 4 5 6 7 8 9 10

If not a "10", what will I do tomorrow to make it closer to a "10"? _____

I ate my frog today: Yes   No   I did my new habit: Yes   No

What Time? _____   What Time? _____

FOR TOMORROW

"Don't judge each day by the harvest you reap, but by the seeds you plant."
Robert Louis Stevenson

DAILY PREVIEW
DAY 75

M T W T F S S

Date: _____

MY PRIMARY OBJECTIVE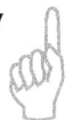

The most important thing I can do today to take me a step closer to my Primary Objective is _____.

The most important thing I can do today to take me a step closer to my Primary Objective is _____.

The most important thing I can do today to take me a step closer to my Primary Objective is _____.

The most important thing I can do today to take me a step closer to my Primary Objective is _____.

My new habit I'm developing (eliminating) is... _____

MORNING THOUGHTS AND INSPIRATIONS

My biggest frog to eat today...
_____

ACTION STEPS FOR TODAY

High Priority
1. _____
2. _____
3. _____

Medium Priority
1. _____
2. _____
3. _____

Low Priority
_____
_____
_____
_____
_____
_____

In which area(s) do I want to improve the most today?

Mental Health

Spiritual Health

Career Health

Physical Health

Social Health

Family Health

Financial Health

Weekly Goal Focus:

DAILY REVIEW
DAY 75

Today I am grateful for...

How was my day? Did I feel good about my performance? What did I learn? Did I have a new insight? What would I do differently?

NOTES AND REFLECTIONS FROM TODAY

What was my energy level today? (lowest to highest) 1 2 3 4 5 6 7 8 9 10

If not a "10", what will I do tomorrow to make it closer to a "10"? _____

I ate my frog today: Yes   No

I did my new habit: Yes   No

What Time? _____

What Time? _____

FOR TOMORROW

"If you want to enjoy the rainbow, be prepared to endure the storm."
Warren Wendel Wiesbe

Life Alchemy 1.0   175

DAILY PREVIEW
DAY 76

M T W T F S S

Date: _____

MY PRIMARY OBJECTIVE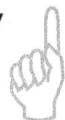

The most important thing I can do today to take me a step closer to my Primary Objective is _____.

The most important thing I can do today to take me a step closer to my Primary Objective is _____.

The most important thing I can do today to take me a step closer to my Primary Objective is _____.

The most important thing I can do today to take me a step closer to my Primary Objective is _____.

My new habit I'm developing (eliminating) is... _____

MORNING THOUGHTS AND INSPIRATIONS

My biggest frog to eat today...
_____

ACTION STEPS FOR TODAY

High Priority
1. _____
2. _____
3. _____

Medium Priority
1. _____
2. _____
3. _____

Low Priority
_____
_____
_____
_____
_____
_____

In which area(s) do I want to improve the most today?

Mental Health

Spiritual Health

Career Health

Physical Health

Social Health

Family Health

Financial Health

Weekly Goal Focus:

DAILY REVIEW
DAY 76

Today I am grateful for...

How was my day? Did I feel good about my performance? What did I learn? Did I have a new insight? What would I do differently?

NOTES AND REFLECTIONS FROM TODAY

What was my energy level today? (lowest to highest) 1 2 3 4 5 6 7 8 9 10

If not a "10", what will I do tomorrow to make it closer to a "10"? _____

I ate my frog today: Yes   No

What Time? _____

I did my new habit: Yes   No

What Time? _____

FOR TOMORROW

"The more you recognize and express gratitude for the things you have, the more things you will have to express gratitude for."

Zig Zigler

DAILY PREVIEW
DAY 77

M T W T F S S

Date: _____

MY PRIMARY OBJECTIVE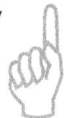

The most important thing I can do today to take me a step closer to my Primary Objective is _____.

The most important thing I can do today to take me a step closer to my Primary Objective is _____.

The most important thing I can do today to take me a step closer to my Primary Objective is _____.

The most important thing I can do today to take me a step closer to my Primary Objective is _____.

My new habit I'm developing (eliminating) is... _____

MORNING THOUGHTS AND INSPIRATIONS

My biggest frog to eat today...
_____

ACTION STEPS FOR TODAY

High Priority
1. _____
2. _____
3. _____

Medium Priority
1. _____
2. _____
3. _____

Low Priority
_____
_____
_____
_____
_____
_____

In which area(s) do I want to improve the most today?

Mental Health

Spiritual Health

Career Health

Physical Health

Social Health

Family Health

Financial Health

Weekly Goal Focus:

DAILY REVIEW
DAY 77

Today I am grateful for...

How was my day? Did I feel good about my performance? What did I learn? Did I have a new insight? What would I do differently?

NOTES AND REFLECTIONS FROM TODAY

What was my energy level today? (lowest to highest) 1 2 3 4 5 6 7 8 9 10

If not a "10", what will I do tomorrow to make it closer to a "10"? _____

I ate my frog today: Yes   No

What Time? _____

I did my new habit: Yes   No

What Time? _____

FOR TOMORROW

"It is never too late to be who you might have been."

George Eliot

Life Alchemy 1.0

WEEKLY CHECK-INS
WEEK 11

The Purpose of the Weekly Check-In is to...

1) Check-in with your progress throughout the week.

2) Re-focus for the upcoming week.

3) Get inspired for the future.

THE CHECK-IN

What have I accomplished since last week? What were the two most important things that I learned this week? Is there anything that I would have done differently? If so, what?

___

What are my wins or victories since last week?

___

What's the highlight (or low-light) of my week?

___

What am I thankful for this week?

___

The place I feel stuck is

___

In which area(s) did I grow the most last week?

Mental Health

Spiritual Health

Career Health

Physical Health

Social Health

Family Health

Financial Health

What was my average energy level for the week?

1 2 3 4 5 6 7 8 9 10

What number do I want it to be next week?

1 2 3 4 5 6 7 8 9 10

How often did you eat your frog?

1 2 3 4 5 6 7

On a 1 - 10 scale, 1 being low and 10 being high, how grateful have I been feeling this last week?

1 2 3 4 5 6 7 8 9 10

How did I do with my new habit building/eliminating?

___

Every week, we will be re-focusing on our future life. So, take a moment and fill this in again. There will be a few questions after you finish.

RE-FOCUS
WEEK 11

If there were no rules, and I could not fail, what would my life be like?

Describe your future life in detail and in writing...

___
___
___
___
___
___
___
___

When you wrote this out again, how did you feel? Were you excited? Were you bored? Did your vision evolve? Was it different than before? Was there more detail or less? Did you even do this exercise? If not, how come?

___
___
___

Look through your future life. Now, fill in the blank...

If I only accomplish _____ next week, my future life would surely come to be.

This is your Primary Objective for the next week.

Take a moment and fill in the days of the week for the next week.

Go on to Day 78 and be amazing!

DAILY PREVIEW
DAY 78

M T W T F S S

Date: _____

MY PRIMARY OBJECTIVE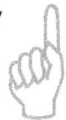

The most important thing I can do today to take me a step closer to my Primary Objective is _____ .

The most important thing I can do today to take me a step closer to my Primary Objective is _____ .

The most important thing I can do today to take me a step closer to my Primary Objective is _____ .

The most important thing I can do today to take me a step closer to my Primary Objective is _____ .

My new habit I'm developing (eliminating) is... _____

MORNING THOUGHTS AND INSPIRATIONS

My biggest frog to eat today...
_____

ACTION STEPS FOR TODAY

High Priority
1. _____
2. _____
3. _____

Medium Priority
1. _____
2. _____
3. _____

Low Priority
_____
_____
_____
_____
_____
_____

In which area(s) do I want to improve the most today?

Mental Health

Spiritual Health

Career Health

Physical Health

Social Health

Family Health

Financial Health

Weekly Goal Focus:

DAILY REVIEW
DAY 78

Today I am grateful for...

_____
_____
_____
_____
_____
_____
_____

How was my day? Did I feel good about my performance? What did I learn? Did I have a new insight? What would I do differently?

_____
_____
_____
_____
_____
_____
_____

NOTES AND REFLECTIONS FROM TODAY

What was my energy level today? (lowest to highest) 1 2 3 4 5 6 7 8 9 10

If not a "10", what will I do tomorrow to make it closer to a "10"? _____

I ate my frog today: Yes   No

What Time? _____

I did my new habit: Yes   No

What Time? _____

FOR TOMORROW

_____
_____
_____
_____

"Be thankful for what you have; you'll end up having more. If you concentrate on what you don't have, you will never, ever have enough."

Oprah Winfrey

Life Alchemy 1.0

DAILY PREVIEW
DAY 79

M T W T F S S

Date: _____

MY PRIMARY OBJECTIVE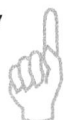

_____

The most important thing I can do today to take me a step closer to my Primary Objective is _____.

The most important thing I can do today to take me a step closer to my Primary Objective is _____.

The most important thing I can do today to take me a step closer to my Primary Objective is _____.

The most important thing I can do today to take me a step closer to my Primary Objective is _____.

My new habit I'm developing (eliminating) is... _____

MORNING THOUGHTS AND INSPIRATIONS

_____

My biggest frog to eat today...
_____

ACTION STEPS FOR TODAY

High Priority
1. _____
2. _____
3. _____

Medium Priority
1. _____
2. _____
3. _____

Low Priority
_____
_____
_____
_____
_____
_____

In which area(s) do I want to improve the most today?

Mental Health

Spiritual Health

Career Health

Physical Health

Social Health

Family Health

Financial Health

Weekly Goal Focus:

DAILY REVIEW
DAY 79

Today I am grateful for...

How was my day? Did I feel good about my performance? What did I learn? Did I have a new insight? What would I do differently?

NOTES AND REFLECTIONS FROM TODAY

What was my energy level today? (lowest to highest) 1 2 3 4 5 6 7 8 9 10

If not a "10", what will I do tomorrow to make it closer to a "10"? _____

I ate my frog today: Yes   No

What Time? _____

I did my new habit: Yes   No

What Time? _____

FOR TOMORROW

"Success is to be measured not so much by the position that one has reached in life as by the obstacles which he has overcome."

Booker T. Washington

Life Alchemy 1.0 **185**

DAILY PREVIEW
DAY 80

M T W T F S S

Date: _____

MY PRIMARY OBJECTIVE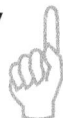

The most important thing I can do today to take me a step closer to my Primary Objective is _____ .

The most important thing I can do today to take me a step closer to my Primary Objective is _____ .

The most important thing I can do today to take me a step closer to my Primary Objective is _____ .

The most important thing I can do today to take me a step closer to my Primary Objective is _____ .

My new habit I'm developing (eliminating) is... _____

MORNING THOUGHTS AND INSPIRATIONS

My biggest frog to eat today...
_____

ACTION STEPS FOR TODAY

High Priority
1. _____
2. _____
3. _____

Medium Priority
1. _____
2. _____
3. _____

Low Priority
_____
_____
_____
_____
_____
_____

In which area(s) do I want to improve the most today?

Mental Health

Spiritual Health

Career Health

Physical Health

Social Health

Family Health

Financial Health

Weekly Goal Focus:

DAILY REVIEW
DAY 80

Today I am grateful for...

How was my day? Did I feel good about my performance? What did I learn? Did I have a new insight? What would I do differently?

NOTES AND REFLECTIONS FROM TODAY

What was my energy level today? (lowest to highest) 1 2 3 4 5 6 7 8 9 10

If not a "10", what will I do tomorrow to make it closer to a "10"? _____

I ate my frog today: Yes   No

I did my new habit: Yes   No

What Time? _____

What Time? _____

FOR TOMORROW

"The greatest glory in living lies not in never falling, but in rising every time we fall."

Nelson Mandela

Life Alchemy 1.0

DAILY PREVIEW
DAY 81

M T W T F S S

Date: _____

MY PRIMARY OBJECTIVE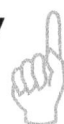

[   ]

The most important thing I can do today to take me a step closer to my Primary Objective is _____.

The most important thing I can do today to take me a step closer to my Primary Objective is _____.

The most important thing I can do today to take me a step closer to my Primary Objective is _____.

The most important thing I can do today to take me a step closer to my Primary Objective is _____.

My new habit I'm developing (eliminating) is... _____

MORNING THOUGHTS AND INSPIRATIONS

My biggest frog to eat today...
_____

ACTION STEPS FOR TODAY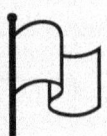

High Priority
1. _____
2. _____
3. _____

Medium Priority
1. _____
2. _____
3. _____

Low Priority
_____
_____
_____
_____
_____
_____

In which area(s) do I want to improve the most today?

Mental Health

Spiritual Health

Career Health

Physical Health

Social Health

Family Health

Financial Health

Weekly Goal Focus:

DAILY REVIEW
DAY 81

Today I am grateful for...

_____
_____
_____
_____
_____
_____
_____
_____

How was my day? Did I feel good about my performance? What did I learn? Did I have a new insight? What would I do differently?

_____
_____
_____
_____
_____
_____
_____
_____

NOTES AND REFLECTIONS FROM TODAY

What was my energy level today? (lowest to highest)   1 2 3 4 5 6 7 8 9 10

If not a "10", what will I do tomorrow to make it closer to a "10"? _____

I ate my frog today: Yes   No

What Time? _____

I did my new habit: Yes   No

What Time? _____

FOR TOMORROW

_____
_____
_____
_____

"If you cannot do great things, do small things in a great way."

Napoleon Hill

Life Alchemy 1.0

DAILY PREVIEW
DAY 82

M T W T F S S

Date: _____

MY PRIMARY OBJECTIVE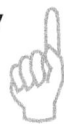

The most important thing I can do today to take me a step closer to my Primary Objective is _____.

The most important thing I can do today to take me a step closer to my Primary Objective is _____.

The most important thing I can do today to take me a step closer to my Primary Objective is _____.

The most important thing I can do today to take me a step closer to my Primary Objective is _____.

My new habit I'm developing (eliminating) is... _____

MORNING THOUGHTS AND INSPIRATIONS

My biggest frog to eat today...
_____

ACTION STEPS FOR TODAY

High Priority
1. _____
2. _____
3. _____

Medium Priority
1. _____
2. _____
3. _____

Low Priority
_____
_____
_____
_____
_____
_____

In which area(s) do I want to improve the most today?

Mental Health

Spiritual Health

Career Health

Physical Health

Social Health

Family Health

Financial Health

Weekly Goal Focus:

DAILY REVIEW
DAY 82

Today I am grateful for...

_____
_____
_____
_____
_____
_____
_____
_____

How was my day? Did I feel good about my performance? What did I learn? Did I have a new insight? What would I do differently?

_____
_____
_____
_____
_____
_____
_____
_____

NOTES AND REFLECTIONS FROM TODAY

What was my energy level today? (lowest to highest)   1 2 3 4 5 6 7 8 9 10

If not a "10", what will I do tomorrow to make it closer to a "10"? _____

I ate my frog today: Yes   No   I did my new habit: Yes   No

What Time? _____   What Time? _____

FOR TOMORROW

_____
_____
_____
_____

"Celebrate what you've accomplished, but raise the bar a little higher each time you succeed."

— *Mia Hamm*

Life Alchemy 1.0

DAILY PREVIEW
DAY 83

M T W T F S S
Date: _____

MY PRIMARY OBJECTIVE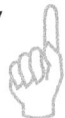

The most important thing I can do today to take me a step closer to my Primary Objective is _____.

The most important thing I can do today to take me a step closer to my Primary Objective is _____.

The most important thing I can do today to take me a step closer to my Primary Objective is _____.

The most important thing I can do today to take me a step closer to my Primary Objective is _____.

My new habit I'm developing (eliminating) is... _____

MORNING THOUGHTS AND INSPIRATIONS

My biggest frog to eat today...
_____

ACTION STEPS FOR TODAY

High Priority
1. _____
2. _____
3. _____

Medium Priority
1. _____
2. _____
3. _____

Low Priority
_____
_____
_____
_____
_____
_____

In which area(s) do I want to improve the most today?

Mental Health
Spiritual Health
Career Health
Physical Health
Social Health
Family Health
Financial Health

Weekly Goal Focus:

DAILY REVIEW
DAY 83

Today I am grateful for...

How was my day? Did I feel good about my performance? What did I learn? Did I have a new insight? What would I do differently?

NOTES AND REFLECTIONS FROM TODAY

What was my energy level today? (lowest to highest)   1 2 3 4 5 6 7 8 9 10

If not a "10", what will I do tomorrow to make it closer to a "10"? _____

I ate my frog today: Yes   No

What Time? _____

I did my new habit: Yes   No

What Time? _____

FOR TOMORROW

"Nothing will work unless you do."
John Wooden

Life Alchemy 1.0

DAILY PREVIEW
DAY 84

M T W T F S S

Date: _____

MY PRIMARY OBJECTIVE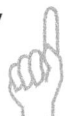

[_____]

The most important thing I can do today to take me a step closer to my Primary Objective is _____.

The most important thing I can do today to take me a step closer to my Primary Objective is _____.

The most important thing I can do today to take me a step closer to my Primary Objective is _____.

The most important thing I can do today to take me a step closer to my Primary Objective is _____.

My new habit I'm developing (eliminating) is... _____

MORNING THOUGHTS AND INSPIRATIONS

My biggest frog to eat today...
_____

ACTION STEPS FOR TODAY

High Priority
1. _____
2. _____
3. _____

Medium Priority
1. _____
2. _____
3. _____

Low Priority
_____
_____
_____
_____
_____
_____
_____

In which area(s) do I want to improve the most today?

Mental Health

Spiritual Health

Career Health

Physical Health

Social Health

Family Health

Financial Health

Weekly Goal Focus:

DAILY REVIEW
DAY 84

Today I am grateful for...

_____
_____
_____
_____
_____
_____
_____

How was my day? Did I feel good about my performance? What did I learn? Did I have a new insight? What would I do differently?

_____
_____
_____
_____
_____
_____
_____

NOTES AND REFLECTIONS FROM TODAY

What was my energy level today? (lowest to highest)   1 2 3 4 5 6 7 8 9 10

If not a "10", what will I do tomorrow to make it closer to a "10"? _____

I ate my frog today: Yes   No   I did my new habit: Yes   No

What Time? _____   What Time? _____

FOR TOMORROW

_____
_____
_____
_____

"Determination that just won't quit – that's what it takes."

— A. J. Foyt

Life Alchemy 1.0

WEEKLY CHECK-INS
WEEK 12

The Purpose of the Weekly Check-In is to...

1) *Check-in with your progress throughout the week.*

2) *Re-focus for the upcoming week.*

3) *Get inspired for the future.*

THE CHECK-IN

What have I accomplished since last week? What were the two most important things that I learned this week? Is there anything that I would have done differently? If so, what?

_____
_____
_____
_____
_____

What are my wins or victories since last week?

_____
_____
_____

What's the highlight (or low-light) of my week?

_____
_____
_____

What am I thankful for this week?

_____
_____
_____

The place I feel stuck is

_____
_____
_____

In which area(s) did I grow the most last week?

Mental Health

Spiritual Health

Career Health

Physical Health

Social Health

Family Health

Financial Health

What was my average energy level for the week?

1 2 3 4 5 6 7 8 9 10

What number do I want it to be next week?

1 2 3 4 5 6 7 8 9 10

How often did you eat your frog?

1 2 3 4 5 6 7

On a 1 - 10 scale, 1 being low and 10 being high, how grateful have I been feeling this last week?

1 2 3 4 5 6 7 8 9 10

How did I do with my new habit building/eliminating?

_____
_____
_____

RE-FOCUS
WEEK 12

Every week, we will be re-focusing on our future life. So, take a moment and fill this in again. There will be a few questions after you finish.

If there were no rules, and I could not fail, what would my life be like?

Describe your future life in detail and in writing...

_____
_____
_____
_____
_____
_____
_____

When you wrote this out again, how did you feel? Were you excited? Were you bored? Did your vision evolve? Was it different than before? Was there more detail or less? Did you even do this exercise? If not, how come?

_____
_____
_____

Look through your future life. Now, fill in the blank...

If I only accomplish _____ next week, my future life would surely come to be.

This is your Primary Objective for the next week.

Take a moment and fill in the days of the week for the next week.

We are coming to the last week of this workbook. If you are finding this process valuable, go to Amazon.com and order Life Alchemy 2.0. This will take you through your next 91 days, and if you do it now, you won't lose any of the momentum you have been building with Life Alchemy 1.0.

Go on to Day 85 and be amazing!

DAILY PREVIEW
DAY 85

M T W T F S S

Date: _____

MY PRIMARY OBJECTIVE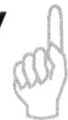

The most important thing I can do today to take me a step closer to my Primary Objective is _____.

The most important thing I can do today to take me a step closer to my Primary Objective is _____.

The most important thing I can do today to take me a step closer to my Primary Objective is _____.

The most important thing I can do today to take me a step closer to my Primary Objective is _____.

My new habit I'm developing (eliminating) is... _____

MORNING THOUGHTS AND INSPIRATIONS

My biggest frog to eat today...
_____

ACTION STEPS FOR TODAY

High Priority
1. _____
2. _____
3. _____

Medium Priority
1. _____
2. _____
3. _____

Low Priority
_____
_____
_____
_____
_____
_____

In which area(s) do I want to improve the most today?

Mental Health

Spiritual Health

Career Health

Physical Health

Social Health

Family Health

Financial Health

Weekly Goal Focus:

DAILY REVIEW
DAY 85

Today I am grateful for...

_____
_____
_____
_____
_____
_____
_____
_____

How was my day? Did I feel good about my performance? What did I learn? Did I have a new insight? What would I do differently?

_____
_____
_____
_____
_____
_____
_____
_____

NOTES AND REFLECTIONS FROM TODAY

What was my energy level today? (lowest to highest)   1 2 3 4 5 6 7 8 9 10

If not a "10", what will I do tomorrow to make it closer to a "10"? _____

I ate my frog today: Yes   No

What Time? _____

I did my new habit: Yes   No

What Time? _____

FOR TOMORROW

_____
_____
_____
_____

"I know the price of success: dedication, hard work, and a devotion to the things you want to see happen."

Frank Lloyd Wright

Life Alchemy 1.0

DAILY PREVIEW
DAY 87

M T W T F S S

Date: _____

MY PRIMARY OBJECTIVE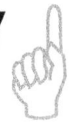

[_____]

The most important thing I can do today to take me a step closer to my Primary Objective is _____ .

The most important thing I can do today to take me a step closer to my Primary Objective is _____ .

The most important thing I can do today to take me a step closer to my Primary Objective is _____ .

The most important thing I can do today to take me a step closer to my Primary Objective is _____ .

My new habit I'm developing (eliminating) is... _____

MORNING THOUGHTS AND INSPIRATIONS

[_____]

My biggest frog to eat today...
_____

ACTION STEPS FOR TODAY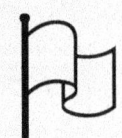

High Priority
1. _____
2. _____
3. _____

Medium Priority
1. _____
2. _____
3. _____

Low Priority
_____
_____
_____
_____
_____
_____

In which area(s) do I want to improve the most today?

Mental Health

Spiritual Health

Career Health

Physical Health

Social Health

Family Health

Financial Health

Weekly Goal Focus:

DAILY REVIEW
DAY 87

Today I am grateful for...

How was my day? Did I feel good about my performance? What did I learn? Did I have a new insight? What would I do differently?

NOTES AND REFLECTIONS FROM TODAY

What was my energy level today? (lowest to highest) 1 2 3 4 5 6 7 8 9 10

If not a "10", what will I do tomorrow to make it closer to a "10"? _____

I ate my frog today: Yes   No   I did my new habit: Yes   No

What Time? _____   What Time? _____

FOR TOMORROW

"All who have accomplished great things have had a great aim; have fixed their gaze on a goal which was high, one which sometimes seemed impossible."

Orison Swett Marden

DAILY PREVIEW
DAY 88

M T W T F S S

Date: _____

MY PRIMARY OBJECTIVE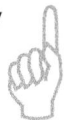

The most important thing I can do today to take me a step closer to my Primary Objective is _____.

The most important thing I can do today to take me a step closer to my Primary Objective is _____.

The most important thing I can do today to take me a step closer to my Primary Objective is _____.

The most important thing I can do today to take me a step closer to my Primary Objective is _____.

My new habit I'm developing (eliminating) is... _____

MORNING THOUGHTS AND INSPIRATIONS

My biggest frog to eat today...
_____

ACTION STEPS FOR TODAY

High Priority
1. _____
2. _____
3. _____

Medium Priority
1. _____
2. _____
3. _____

Low Priority
_____
_____
_____
_____
_____
_____

In which area(s) do I want to improve the most today?

Mental Health

Spiritual Health

Career Health

Physical Health

Social Health

Family Health

Financial Health

Weekly Goal Focus:

DAILY REVIEW
DAY 88

Today I am grateful for...

_____
_____
_____
_____
_____
_____
_____
_____

How was my day? Did I feel good about my performance? What did I learn? Did I have a new insight? What would I do differently?

_____
_____
_____
_____
_____
_____
_____
_____

NOTES AND REFLECTIONS FROM TODAY

What was my energy level today? (lowest to highest)   1 2 3 4 5 6 7 8 9 10

If not a "10", what will I do tomorrow to make it closer to a "10"? _____

I ate my frog today: Yes   No

What Time? _____

I did my new habit: Yes   No

What Time? _____

"Shallow men believe in luck. Strong men believe in cause and effect."
Ralph Waldo Emerson

FOR TOMORROW

_____
_____
_____
_____

Life Alchemy 1.0

DAILY PREVIEW
DAY 89

M T W T F S S

Date: _____

MY PRIMARY OBJECTIVE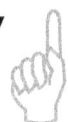

The most important thing I can do today to take me a step closer to my Primary Objective is _____.

The most important thing I can do today to take me a step closer to my Primary Objective is _____.

The most important thing I can do today to take me a step closer to my Primary Objective is _____.

The most important thing I can do today to take me a step closer to my Primary Objective is _____.

My new habit I'm developing (eliminating) is... _____

MORNING THOUGHTS AND INSPIRATIONS

My biggest frog to eat today...
_____

ACTION STEPS FOR TODAY

High Priority
1. _____
2. _____
3. _____

Medium Priority
1. _____
2. _____
3. _____

Low Priority
_____
_____
_____
_____
_____
_____

In which area(s) do I want to improve the most today?

Mental Health

Spiritual Health

Career Health

Physical Health

Social Health

Family Health

Financial Health

Weekly Goal Focus:

DAILY REVIEW
DAY 89

Today I am grateful for...
_____
_____
_____
_____
_____
_____
_____
_____

How was my day? Did I feel good about my performance? What did I learn? Did I have a new insight? What would I do differently?
_____
_____
_____
_____
_____
_____
_____

NOTES AND REFLECTIONS FROM TODAY

What was my energy level today? (lowest to highest)   1 2 3 4 5 6 7 8 9 10

If not a "10", what will I do tomorrow to make it closer to a "10"? _____

I ate my frog today: Yes   No

What Time? _____

I did my new habit: Yes   No

What Time? _____

"Winning is a habit. Unfortunately, so is losing."

Vince Lombardi

FOR TOMORROW
_____
_____
_____
_____

Life Alchemy 1.0

DAILY PREVIEW
DAY 90

M T W T F S S

Date: _____

MY PRIMARY OBJECTIVE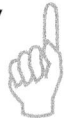

[_____]

The most important thing I can do today to take me a step closer to my Primary Objective is _____.

The most important thing I can do today to take me a step closer to my Primary Objective is _____.

The most important thing I can do today to take me a step closer to my Primary Objective is _____.

The most important thing I can do today to take me a step closer to my Primary Objective is _____.

My new habit I'm developing (eliminating) is... _____

MORNING THOUGHTS AND INSPIRATIONS

My biggest frog to eat today...
_____

ACTION STEPS FOR TODAY

High Priority
1. _____
2. _____
3. _____

Medium Priority
1. _____
2. _____
3. _____

Low Priority
_____
_____
_____
_____
_____
_____

In which area(s) do I want to improve the most today?

Mental Health

Spiritual Health

Career Health

Physical Health

Social Health

Family Health

Financial Health

Weekly Goal Focus:

DAILY REVIEW
DAY 90

Today I am grateful for...

_____
_____
_____
_____
_____
_____
_____

How was my day? Did I feel good about my performance? What did I learn? Did I have a new insight? What would I do differently?

_____
_____
_____
_____
_____
_____
_____

NOTES AND REFLECTIONS FROM TODAY

What was my energy level today? (lowest to highest) 1 2 3 4 5 6 7 8 9 10

If not a "10", what will I do tomorrow to make it closer to a "10"? _____

I ate my frog today: Yes   No

What Time? _____

I did my new habit: Yes   No

What Time? _____

FOR TOMORROW

_____
_____
_____
_____

"Many of life's failures are people who did not realize how close they were to success when they gave up."

Thomas Alva Edison

Life Alchemy 1.0

DAILY PREVIEW
DAY 91

M T W T F S S

Date: _____

MY PRIMARY OBJECTIVE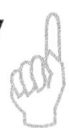

The most important thing I can do today to take me a step closer to my Primary Objective is _____ .

The most important thing I can do today to take me a step closer to my Primary Objective is _____ .

The most important thing I can do today to take me a step closer to my Primary Objective is _____ .

The most important thing I can do today to take me a step closer to my Primary Objective is _____ .

My new habit I'm developing (eliminating) is... _____

MORNING THOUGHTS AND INSPIRATIONS

My biggest frog to eat today...
_____

ACTION STEPS FOR TODAY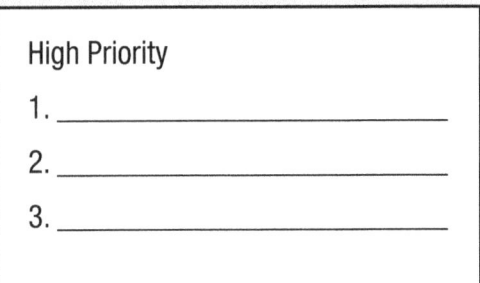

High Priority
1. _____
2. _____
3. _____

Medium Priority
1. _____
2. _____
3. _____

Low Priority
_____
_____
_____
_____
_____
_____

In which area(s) do I want to improve the most today?

Mental Health

Spiritual Health

Career Health

Physical Health

Social Health

Family Health

Financial Health

Weekly Goal Focus:

DAILY REVIEW
DAY 91

Today I am grateful for...

How was my day? Did I feel good about my performance? What did I learn? Did I have a new insight? What would I do differently?

NOTES AND REFLECTIONS FROM TODAY

What was my energy level today? (lowest to highest) 1 2 3 4 5 6 7 8 9 10

If not a "10", what will I do tomorrow to make it closer to a "10"? _____

I ate my frog today: Yes   No

I did my new habit: Yes   No

What Time? _____

What Time? _____

FOR TOMORROW

"It is not your aptitude, but your attitude, that determines your altitude."

Zig Zigler

Life Alchemy 1.0

WEEKLY CHECK-INS
WEEK 13

The Purpose of the Weekly Check-In is to...

1) *Check-in with your progress throughout the week.*

2) *Re-focus for the upcoming week.*

3) *Get inspired for the future.*

THE CHECK-IN

What have I accomplished since last week? What were the two most important things that I learned this week? Is there anything that I would have done differently? If so, what?

_____
_____
_____
_____
_____

What are my wins or victories since last week?

_____
_____
_____

What's the highlight (or low-light) of my week?

_____
_____
_____

What am I thankful for this week?

_____
_____
_____

The place I feel stuck is

_____
_____
_____

In which area(s) did I grow the most last week?

Mental Health

Spiritual Health

Career Health

Physical Health

Social Health

Family Health

Financial Health

What was my average energy level for the week?

1 2 3 4 5 6 7 8 9 10

What number do I want it to be next week?

1 2 3 4 5 6 7 8 9 10

How often did you eat your frog?

1 2 3 4 5 6 7

On a 1 - 10 scale, 1 being low and 10 being high, how grateful have I been feeling this last week?

1 2 3 4 5 6 7 8 9 10

How did I do with my new habit building/eliminating?

_____
_____
_____

RE-FOCUS
WEEK 13

Every week, we will be re-focusing on our future life. So, take a moment and fill this in again. There will be a few questions after you finish.

If there were no rules, and I could not fail, what would my life be like?

Describe your future life in detail and in writing...

_____
_____
_____
_____
_____
_____
_____

When you wrote this out again, how did you feel? Were you excited? Were you bored? Did your vision evolve? Was it different than before? Was there more detail or less? Did you even do this exercise? If not, how come?

_____
_____
_____

Look through your future life. Now, fill in the blank...

If I only accomplish _____ next week, my future life would surely come to be.

This is your Primary Objective for the next week.

Now What?

Life Alchemy 1.0

CONGRATULATE YOURSELF!

You put in the time. You defined your dream life. You focused on your dream and you took action. Either you are living your dream life right now, or you are a lot closer to achieving it than you were just 3 months ago.
Way to go!

If you found value in this process, go to Amazon.com and buy Life Alchemy 2.0. This will take you through your next 3 months. In the meantime, keep your momentum going. While you are waiting for Life Alchemy 2.0 to arrive, download a few daily templates at www.lifealchemybook.com and print them out. By now you have created an awesome new habit of daily journaling that you definitely do not want to break.

Also, tell others about Life Alchemy 1.0. Can you imagine a whole world of people taking action towards their dreams? How cool would that be? Buy one for a loved one today. By the way, if someone bought this one for you, make sure to thank them and let them know how you have been able to improve your life with this little workbook.

Once again, *WAY TO GO!*

ABOUT THE AUTHOR

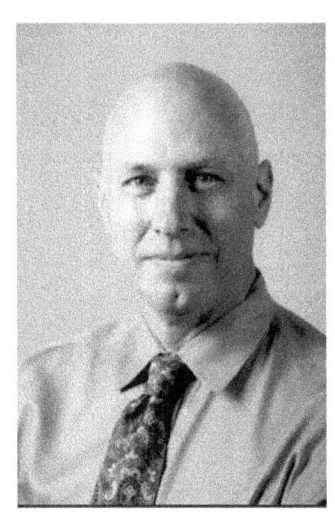

Dr. Dale Ellwein is an author, lecturer and wellness lifestyle specialist. He received his doctorate in Chiropractic from Life Chiropractic College West in Hayward, California, in 1991, and did advance studies with Dr. James L. Chestnut, earning his Chiropractic Wellness Professional Certification. His book, *Dear Oprah: The Health Book for Everyone*, is a staple for those who care about their health.

Dr. Ellwein inspires people of all ages to achieve peak performance, focus, mental acuity, and amazing health. He teaches simple, proven systems that inspire his patients to eat, move and think in ways that support their longevity and vital, healing nature.

Using the essential combination of lifestyle management and advanced chiropractic care, Dr. Ellwein has helped thousands of individuals overcome aches, pains, and diseases, and improve their overall quality of life. His proven program has been shown to restore health and healing in the bodies of his patients—often leading to long, inspired, joy-filled lives.

Dr. Ellwein practices in Southern California, where he lives with his wife, Barbara, two children, three dogs and six chickens. He conducts extensive talks on optimum performance, health and longevity, and several of his talks, videos, and articles can be found on the internet.

For more information on Dr. Dale Ellwein, go to www.thedoctorofthefuture.com.

www.ingramcontent.com/pod-product-compliance
Lightning Source LLC
Chambersburg PA
CBHW080540170426
43195CB00016B/2632